Moments in Quantative

:h

Hilary Byrne-Armstrong PhD, MSc(Hons), GradDipSocEd,
GradDipPty
Centre for Critical Psychology, University of Western Sydney, New South
Wales, Australia

Joy Higgs PhD, MPHEd, GradDipPty, BSc
Centre for Professional Education Advancement, Faculty of Health
Sciences, The University of Sydney, New South Wales, Australia

Debbie Horsfall PhD, MA, BEd
School of Sociology and Justice Studies, University of Western Sydney,
New South Wales, Australia

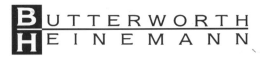

BUTTERWORTH
HEINEMANN

OXFORD AUCKLAND BOSTON JOHANNESBURG MELBOURNE NEW DELHI

Butterworth-Heinemann
Linacre House, Jordan Hill, Oxford OX2 8DP
225 Wildwood Avenue, Woburn, MA 01801-2041
A division of Reed Educational and Professional Publishing Ltd

℞   A member of the Reed Elsevier plc group

First published 2001

British Library Cataloguing in Publication Data
A catalogue record for this book in available from the British Library

Library of Congress Cataloguing in Publication Data
A catalogue record for this book is available from the Library of Congress

ISBN 0 7506 5159 8

For information on all Butterworth-Heinemann publications visit our
website at www.bh.com

Typeset by Keyword Typesetting Services, Wallington and Great Yarmouth
Printed and bound in Great Britain by Biddles Ltd, Guildford and King's Lynn

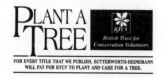

FOR EVERY TITLE THAT WE PUBLISH, BUTTERWORTH-HEINEMANN
WILL PAY FOR BTCV TO PLANT AND CARE FOR A TREE.

Contents

Contributors

Hilary Byrne-Armstrong PhD, MSc(Hons), GradDipSocEd, DipPhty
School of Critical Social Sciences, University of Western Sydney, Hawkesbury, New South Wales, Australia

Moira Carmody PhD, BSW, GradDipEd
School of Sociology and Justice Studies, University of Western Sydney, Hawkesbury, New South Wales, Australia

Heather D'Cruz BSW, MSW, PhD
School of Social Inquiry, Deakin University, Geelong, Victoria, Australia

Mary M Day PhD, MCom(Hons), BBus
Department of Accounting and Finance, University of Wollongong, New South Wales, Australia

Alma Fleet PhD
Institute of Early Childhood, Macquarie University, New South Wales, Australia

Charles Higgs MSocEcol, BSurv
Centre for Professional Education Advancement, Faculty of Health Sciences, The University of Sydney, New South Wales, Australia

Joy Higgs PhD, MPHEd, GradDipPhty, BSc
Faculty of Health Sciences, The University of Sydney, Lidcombe, New South Wales, Australia

Susan Holland PhD, MEd, DipEd, BA
Faculty of Community Services, Education and Social Sciences, Edith Cowan University, Mount Lawley, Western Australia, Australia

Debbie Horsfall PhD, MA, BEd
School of Sociology and Justice Studies, University of Western Sydney, New South Wales, Australia

Virginia Kaufman Hall PhD, MAppSc, BA, DipEd
Human Centred Solutions, Dickson, Australian Capital Territory, Australia

Barbara Leigh PhD
Institute for International Studies, University of Technology, Sydney, Broadway, New South Wales, Australia

Lindy McAllister MA(Hons), BSpThy
School of Community Health, Charles Sturt University, Albury, New South Wales, Australia

Martin Mulligan PhD
Social Ecology, University of Western Sydney, New South Wales, Australia

Catherine Patterson PhD, MEd
Institute of Early Childhood, Macquarie University, New South Wales, Australia

Judy Pinn MEd, BA, DipEd
University of Western Sydney, Hawkesbury, New South Wales, Australia

David Smith PhD, BA(Hons)
Dept of Teaching and Curriculum Studies, Faculty of Education, The University of Sydney, New South Wales, Australia

Susan M Thompson PhD, MTCP, BA(Hons), DipEd, MRAPI
Faculty of the Built Environment, University of New South Wales, Sydney, New South Wales, Australia

Preface

Research is often presented as a coherent, carefully constructed, linear and systematic activity. As experienced qualitative researchers, we question this representation. Research is complex, often chaotic, sometimes messy, even conflictual, full of critical moments that disrupt our process, moments when our inner voices or the outer world, with its structures and conventions, intrude. In this book we speak the often unspeakable, give voice to the critical moments often sanitized from research processes; critical moments that are not written into research documents, or even acknowledged as part of the everyday life of any researcher. The aim of this book is to 'sing up', or illuminate, these critical moments.

This book is intended for researchers, research students, supervisors and reviewers. It is the product of research and scholarship. The authors have explored the critical moments of qualitative research that they and others have experienced or researched. We invite readers to reflect on these writings and to continue, with us, to develop and explore the endless possibilities, as well as the real-world dilemmas of qualitative research.

We would like to thank our team of authors and peer reviewers for their scholarly, creative and critical input to this project, facilitated through the Centre for Professional Education Advancement at The University of Sydney. We also wish to pay special tribute to Joan Rosenthal for her invaluable role in facilitating the process of collaboration and review of this book.

Hilary Byrne-Armstrong, Joy Higgs and Debbie Horsfall

Section One

Knowledge and practice

1

Researching critical moments

Debbie Horsfall, Hilary Byrne-Armstrong and Joy Higgs

The tension that we need to maintain between the rich diffuse, complex character of everyday life and the ways our literatures organise and symbolise its buzzing confusions sustains the moral tenor of our work. (Grumet, 1990, p. 339)

As a researcher, student or supervisor, do you ever wonder where the self-doubt, messiness, creativity and complexity of doing research disappears?

- *As a researcher:*
  When you read others' research reports, do you feel that you are the only one having difficulty doing research?
  Do you wonder how to manage difficult relationships which, though second-ary to your research, are getting in the way?
  Do you ever wonder whether what you are involved in is research, because you seem to spend more time negotiating with agencies, colleagues and structures than doing your research?

- *As a supervisor:*
  Have you ever searched for something to give your students to reassure them when they are about to give up on their research?
  How do you assist your students to negotiate conflicting methodologies?

We did, hence this book. When reading research reports one rarely hears about any of the above situations. The dominant convention is to sanitize research reporting. In the light of this tendency anyone could be forgiven for believing that extremely sophisticated and competent computers conduct most research. Removing research from the context of the relationships in which it is embedded mystifies it and places it in an ivory tower that can be reached only by the anointed. That research is a part of everyday life is disguised, maintaining the barrier between everyday living and research. The effect of this on potential new researchers is not helpful; indeed, it is often obstructive. Rather than debate why this conspiracy of silence might exist, this book seeks to provide concrete examples of how people are already challenging this barrier to illuminating the reality of research. There is edginess regarding 'telling it as it is', admitting dilemmas, mistakes, difficult relationships, struggles, or less than perfect practices of research. However, if these things are not openly talked about we cannot learn from them, and others coming after us are discouraged when they encounter their own research realities. This book opens the space for researchers to talk about and learn practical strategies for doing their research in the face of often obstructive conventions.

Some rules and conventions are sensible and useful. Others are oppressive. It is important to be aware of the conventions and the rationale for their existence, in order to negotiate them. This negotiation may be passionate, messy, creative, or filled with crises and confrontations. It can be a passive form of resistance or a rational form of bargaining, or even walking away. It is this process of negotiation that shapes the identities and ethics of all involved in the research.

For this book, people were asked to speak about the messy, unspoken, complex, and disturbing moments in their research processes. We called them critical moments. Critical moments are those times when researchers are impelled to negotiate between the theories and conventions about research and their lived experience of it. Critical moments tell us the truth of the research process.

We faced a number of critical moments ourselves as editors of this publication on research. The first two publishers we approached turned us down. One wanted a 'how to' style of book, which we were seeking to avoid; the second found the topic too adventurous. We faced the challenge of whether to make the book more orthodox or keep seeking a creative publisher. We clearly had to choose the latter course. In our current publisher we found kindred spirits, people prepared to look at research publications with fresh eyes. Another critical moment was encountered as we proposed the task and style of writing in this book to the authors. Some authors faced the 'bare-all' task with alacrity, while others needed some encouragement to put aside the constraints of sanitized writing often expected of them. We spent some time debating the level of explanation needed for novice readers compared to the degree of reflection and revelation that would be more accessible to experienced researchers.

We chose the metaphor 'critical moments' to represent those experiences that are not usually written into research documents, or even formally acknowledged as part of the everyday life of every researcher. The authors were asked to consider challenging research as a sanitized process in the following ways:

- acknowledging critical moments as important intellectual springboards
- giving voice to the often silenced identity of the researcher
- recognizing that critical moments are re-authoring opportunities
- making research less mysterious and more accessible for new researchers
- giving voice to silenced stories
- challenging the frequent presentation of research as a neat, systematic process
- producing other discourses and knowledge(s) about research and therefore creating more spaces for people and researchers to inhabit.

For the organization of the book, we used three guiding metaphors. The choice of metaphors organized the content into three interwoven themes: methodological issues (lost in space and time), relationship issues (the full Monty), and structural issues (glass ceilings and brick walls).

Methodological issues: lost in space and time

This first section emerged from the question, 'How does one negotiate the research convention of a single methodology in the face of the everyday experience of multiple methodologies?'. Trying to fit the lived experience of researching to this convention can, for many, lead to a feeling of bewilderment, of being lost and confused. Methods and methodology are not always singular, *a priori*, fixed and unchanging. The chapters in this section tell a different story. Methodology and method often emerge, shifting and changing as knowledge is produced. Methodology may be like a patchwork quilt, created and stitched up during the research.

Heather d'Cruz stitches together the work of Foucault, Bourdieu and Potter, feminist sociology, identity politics and critical discourse analysis in her investigation of meanings and identities in reports of child protection workers on childhood abuse. She talks about the factors, such as place and time, which influenced the development of methodology, commenting that her methodological choice was also connected to her identity and subjectivity as a researcher, confirming that the researcher and the research are intertwined. Heather uses a metaphor of a lens, fracturing it and moving between the lens as microscope or camera and the lens as a pair of glasses or binoculars. This interposition of a lens represents a disruption in the research practices that constitute the researched as simply objects of research, and the researcher as the subject. The disruption enables both the researcher and the researched to voice the reality that everybody moves between subject/object, knower/known, as they are changed by the research process.

The second chapter in this section visits the old, but still influential argument between positivist and post-positivist researchers. Many of the questions of new researchers are answered, and strategies are explored for negotiating with the rules and regulations constructing how we are 'allowed' to do research. While many view this negotiation as a struggle, Charles Higgs and Lindy McAllister, playfully using the metaphor of a space cadet, capture the excitement, wonder and pleasure which new researchers also experience as they navigate through unknown territories – boldly going where no person has gone before! The understanding of 'new worlds' emerges from the exploratory negotiations, expressed as a conversation between the authors, who take the roles of novice and experienced methodological space cadets. For both novice and experienced researchers, this chapter provides a clear and useful discussion of the principles of qualitative and interpretive research, and a comprehensive bibliography.

The next chapter, from Joy Higgs, looks at the different standpoints in qualitative research. Using five metaphors – being lost in space and time, framing the research journey, dancing on the carpet, illuminating the phenomenon, and conversing with peers and sages – this chapter relates research to a journey in space and time where these five critical moments require the researcher to learn how to chart directions and standpoints to achieve a successful journey. The challenges and opportunities in each of these moments are explored. So, too, we are reminded of the dangers of unauthentic research, inadequate transfer from the terminology and restrictions of quantitative research, and failing to set high standards, thus earning justified criticism from quantitative researchers.

The last chapter in this section explores the crisis in which one can find oneself when doing a large project such as a PhD. What happens when the reading and researching undertaken mean that one's initial proposal and intellectual stance is no longer valid? Hilary Byrne-Armstrong found herself constructing a very different thesis from the one she set out to produce. In the process of doing this she re-authored herself from one who researched others' learning transitions to recognizing her learning as inextricably woven with theirs; from one who researched collaboratively to one who challenged these same methods on the grounds of ethics. The negotiation between everyday life, theory and practice became her knowing and being dilemmas, and kept the material alive and embodied. Her challenge, or critical moment, was to write a thesis that demonstrated this.

Relationship issues: the full Monty

This section invites the writers to 'bare all' as it focuses on the numerous relationships that the researcher navigates, including the relationship with oneself as a writer and researcher, the relationship with supervisors and examiners, and the relationships with families and friends. Research is normally constructed as a singular and isolated activity. The fact that researchers are also people with families and friends, with social and cultural heritages and personal histories, remains hidden in most research. Yet these everyday relationships and our navigation of them often have a significant impact on the type of research we do and how we do it. This, of course, works both ways.

All researching involves writing, yet the embodied act of writing is kept hidden in research reports. The first chapter in this section is an exploration of the struggle of a researcher to find her voice as a writer. Debbie Horsfall explores writing/researching from the aspect of her social and cultural history. She shifts the focus from writing research as a re-presentation of facts, of telling 'the truth', to one of constructing a story, negotiating the many truths that often become apparent as one researches. This shift, she argues, makes more transparent the social practices that shape and often silence many of our voices as researchers/writers. This she regards as a political act (a subversive practice), one in which the researcher steps into her shoes as author and authority. Understanding 'writer's block' not just as a pathological response of the writer but also as socially constructed enables the researcher/writer to say what needs to be said.

Arguably, one of the most important relationships to researchers undertaking a research degree is that between the student and supervisor. Alma Fleet, Susan Holland, Barbara Leigh and Catherine Patterson write of their own and other women's experiences as students doing research degrees. Their central idea is that this relationship cannot ever be robust because of the power differential and the length of time it has to be sustained. Using metaphors of the changing moods of the sea, they describe the experience of women as they negotiate the process of attaining a higher degree. The support that many women found to keep going and complete their degrees came not from officially sanctioned relationships, but from family and colleagues. In the experiences they recount, the social practices of the institution still reinforce gender stereotypes that are dominating and oppressive. However, the authors are also careful to describe the exhilaration, wonder and sense of achievement as well as the struggles involved, confirming the sense of agency that is often gained through these adventures.

The next chapter explores the idea of collaboration in the face of the power/knowledge relationship in research. Hilary Byrne-Armstrong tells stories from her research to illustrate the changing meanings of a series of events that led her from an initially enthusiastic humanist inquiry to a bewildered and critical view of the collaborative action research process. The stories are a vivid account of how the power/knowledge relationship can interrupt the research process. They are told as instances illustrating how ideas such as collaboration disguise the power inherent in the researching process because of the complex, competing and different interests and agendas. Negotiating these agendas, rather than keeping them silenced and sanitized, is part of the collaborative researching process. Her initial response was to explore and develop a reflexive methodology that included the many different voices and competing agendas in the research process. This eventually changed her direction in research and her position as a researcher, leading her away from co-researching with people to co-researching (with or without people) with the collective interpretations and narratives that constitute people's lives.

Virginia Kaufman Hall, an experienced skilled social researcher, reflects on working as a qualitative researcher with government departments in Australia. Her passion is to use her skills to influence public policy and programme development, a challenge, she feels, in this age of economic rationalism. Using a storytelling approach, Virginia details how qualitative research can be and is used as a valuable tool for change, and how the social researcher concerned with social justice can negotiate economic rationalism, which dominates departmental language and current decision-making. Virginia details the principles of respectful inquiry that underpin her research approach in working with, rather than on, people. This way of working, she argues, enables the social researcher to tell a better story of the society in which we live and provide a fuller understanding of why we experience the world as we do. It is this level of detail, which comes from people's stories, that can powerfully affect public policy and decision makers in government departments.

As the previous chapters show, great care is needed to negotiate the research relationship. The supervisor can feel extremely exposed, walking the fine line between being a voyeur, a therapist and a teacher/supervisor. David Smith reflects on these issues as he writes about his development as a supervisor, learning about the substantive content areas of students, learning about communication, and learning about himself. He recognizes that much of his skill as a supervisor has emerged from purposeful reflection on his own experiences as a supervisee. This skill involves negotiating the shifting supervisor/teacher/student relationship. Sometimes one will be a coach and mentor, at other times a gatekeeper, and at yet other times a peer researcher. What is ultimately revealed is that supervision can be seen as a privilege and a gift.

Martin Mulligan writes of the critical moments when life, work and research collide. In spite of the dominant story telling us that our lives are compartmentalized and separate, this is not how most of us live/work; we are all embedded in many relationships which influence the lives we lead and the work we do. Rather than seeking to keep these relationships hidden, Martin suggests that we blur the boundaries between life, work and research, and open up the possibility for more meaningful research as we allow these other influences to be heard. This, he suggests, means negotiating the relationship between control and chaos. Moving between order/ predictability and chaos/complexity can enable sparks of creativity and passion to fly, research and the researcher to come alive.

Structural issues: glass ceilings and brick walls

The last section describes the structural constraints, regulations and politics that we know get in our way as researchers, and which become more obstructive if they remain invisible. Making them visible is important, not because we necessarily want to tear them down but because it is how we negotiate these constraints that determines our success or otherwise as researchers.

What could be called dramatic disruptions and monstrous practices are a welcome relief. They model how we can resist being totally captured by the dominant story of researching. Mary Day's poem, in the context of academia, is one such courageous practice, which clearly names the structures and everyday social practices she has experienced as oppressive and silencing in her work. The poem speaks for itself through its artistic merit, and is a good example of creativity emerging out of critical moments in research.

Susan Thompson has also shattered some of the panes of glass and pushed out many of the bricks. She writes unapologetically about her negotiation with the rigid walls of prejudice as a qualitative researcher in urban planning. Carefully, she describes the ethical position she is taking and then presents cogent arguments to the mainstream voices that challenge her work. Brick by brick she dismantles each of these arguments, from feminist and qualitative research positions. Many of the arguments portray the prejudice and narrow-mindedness of the 'fortress' which is positivist research. Susan's chapter provides an excellent resource and inspiration for new researchers. Her voice is strong and her confidence is helpful in the face of intimidatory practices such as many qualitative researchers continue to encounter. Despite the fact that we would like to think that this is an old argument, Susan's chapter reminds us that for some people in some contexts it is not only highly influential, but alive and kicking.

Often intimidatory and silencing social practices are rendered invisible, kept quiet, and in so doing the skills and lessons learnt from dealing with them are not passed on to our fellow travellers. Moira Carmody's chapter makes the invisible visible. Moira is a qualitative researcher who has worked for many years in the area of sexual violence and public policy; her work represents negotiating a triple brick wall. Within the literary convention of a play, each scene captures a critical moment negotiated in completing a recent research project. Played out are intimidation, denial, group relationship issues, and the exercise of power for both productive and dominating ends. Moira explores the links between the activities of research, political action and ethical practice. The convention of a play illustrates the way in which, when we negotiate these critical moments, creativity can come to the fore.

Negotiating critical moments often gives rise to the creative edge that is required to present qualitative research. Judy Pinn uses a number of stories from her practice as a researcher and supervisor to illustrate the crisis of representation and how people have negotiated this creatively. She shows that the critical moments in any research can lead to forms of creative representations. Wrestling with these critical moments, be they crises of confidence, writer's block, or intimidation (either overt or covert), can open the space for people to act otherwise, to reinvent and reinscribe practices, to do something they might otherwise not have thought of. Judy suggests that often we do not realize how subversive and disruptive this 'doing otherwise' can be. The chapter shows, both theoretically and practically, how a number of researchers simultaneously conform to and transgress dominant research conventions.

The final chapter looks at critical moments (many times presented as brick walls or experimental design frameworks imposed by dominant traditions) encountered by qualitative research examiners. These critical moments often appear in the form of ethical dilemmas where prospective examiners are faced with decisions relating to assessing their own capacity to do justice to the given research strategy and topic, and to balancing the expectations of the institution and the research product. Joy examines the frameworks different research paradigms provide for researchers and examiners alike, the standards that demonstrate quality and that special, intangible essence that characterizes the outstanding thesis.

Reflections

In reflecting on the chapters our authors submitted, we asked ourselves the following questions:

- What themes or knowledge(s) seeped in throughout the collection?
- What crept through the cracks of the text, heralding the unexpected?
- What is the emergent spirit of the collection?
- Were there commonalities in our authors' experiences that would help to add to the discourses of qualitative research?

Our reading of the chapters identified six themes: resistance, pleasure, rites of passage, ethics, rigour and reframing.

Resistance

The resistance theme was so prominent that we asked ourselves, 'Did we produce a resistance discourse in the framing of our book?'. The answer is probably 'yes'. In the original outline sent to contributors, we questioned the construction of research as 'coherent, carefully constructed, linear and systematic'. Implicit in this was the contention that this depiction was not accurate and that we needed to resist it. Our invitation read as though we were recruiting other resistance workers! This in turn shaped the practice of the writers. Resistance is present in most of the chapters, but is epitomized in Chapters 3, 13 and 16. Most of the chapters describe a struggle – a struggle with relationships, with methodologies or with structures. There is a tension in making these struggles visible in a book such as this. Our aim is to encourage researchers, not to scare them off! The struggle seemingly inherent in doing qualitative social research can often be painful if not dangerous.

Also apparent in this collection is the realization that struggle is not necessarily a negative phenomenon. It can be the creative process of moving outside the rigidity of the boxes we inhabit to create new identities for ourselves and new practices that may be useful for others. Like snakes we outgrow our skin, struggling to free ourselves of what is, to become what might be, in the ongoing challenge with life.

Pleasure

The disruption of the resistance discourse was present in the many instances of pleasure that people demonstrated in their practices. There was pleasure in finding a voice; pleasure in writing and creativity; pleasure in the solitary nature of the writing process; pleasure in the rites of passage to greater understandings; pleasure in creating and recreating direction; pleasure in finally getting one's head around theory; pleasure at reinventing ourselves as competent researchers; pleasure in setting our own high standards and reaching them; pleasure because research provides, in many examples, a cliff edge at which to test ourselves to see what we are capable of, and to wonder what will happen if . . . ? The pleasure in critical moments peeked through the nooks and crannies of most of the chapters.

In the face of a problem-saturated world, the pleasurable stories about research need to be told alongside the struggles and resistances. After all, many of us who embarked on an initial and single research project are still, many years later, researching. There must be pleasure and satisfaction in it somewhere. The stories from our authors confirm this. Next time, we might frame a book in terms of the pleasurable moments in research!

Rites of passage

Rites of passage are the process for facilitating transitions in social life from one identity and position to another (van Gennep, 1960). Researching is a rite of passage. This was particularly evident in the chapters that referred to the task of getting a PhD. It is most clearly reflected in the relationship section – the full Monty.

The rite of passage metaphor is often silenced in collaborative research by the emphasis on equality, sharing and co-researching. However, collaboration, as can be seen in Chapter 8, disguises power, and often makes research initiators shy about their position and the individual achievement inherent in managing a research project (or managing a postgraduate student successfully). To use the metaphor of researching as a rite of passage helps these more individual endeavours and achievements become public. It enables researchers to acknowledge their intellectual achievements, to feel proud about sustaining relationships and knowing that they have produced knowledge(s). In other words, it frames the research as a personal and subjective process as well as an objective task.

Finally, research provides fertile ground for what Foucault (1980) called 'refusing what we are', for creating ourselves anew in the face of the dominating forces in our culture. One of the joys of research is learning to play the discursive field, finding agency within and against dominant forms of identity and creating new identities. Many would consider this a self-centred aim. Most of our contributors recognized the power positions they had attained by traversing the rite of passage that is research. In this recognition, they acknowledged the politics of research and their privilege. They also showed themselves as models and mentors for others, as trailblazers who could open the space for those who come later.

Ethics

The moral tenor of research is maintained as we hold the tension between our everyday lives and the way in which we are organized by research conventions. The ethical practices of our contributors are demonstrated throughout the book in the reflexivity apparent in each chapter. The reflexive interaction with the world is an ethical interaction. For example, David's recognition of himself as a supervisor shaped by his own supervisory experiences illustrates ethical practice and reflexivity. Reflexivity is also present when Alma and co-authors discuss the social practices shaping the behaviour of supervisors. It is present when Hilary recognizes that her desire as a research initiator to be fully collaborative will always be negated by the competitive discourse. It is present in Debbie's recognition that her voice as a writer is shaped by her positioning in society and culture, in Judy's understanding of the intersection of individual and cultural forces, in Moira's refusal to be 'shut up', in Joy's exploration of the thesis examiner's role, and in Heather's acknowledgment that her upbringing contributed to her choice of methodology.

It is important in this age of rampant reflexivity that none of our writers used this as an excuse not to act. Perusing the writing of their actions, we realize once again that opening the space for multiple knowledge(s) can lead to a space of infinite creativity and possibility. The more stories we read, the more research we did on this topic, the more we realized that the interlocking multiplicity of critical moments, rather than paralysing us, heightened our excitement and enthusiasm for the possibilities of the research process. These possibilities are not ephemeral. They are material, real and *already present* in everyday life. Knowing this can enable people to act in multiple ways and, we hope, enable new researchers to see where they can insert their own voices and practices in the business of producing knowledge that is called research.

Rigour

This word is usually associated with positivist research; it sends many qualitative researchers quivering into the corner or turning to more compatible terms. We want to reclaim it; indeed, to liberate it. Our work as researchers had increasingly focused on difference, complexity and conflict as being the compost of everyday life. As all good composters know, compost has to be maintained at a certain degree of heat, be constantly moved around and added to, and is inhabited by many invisible creatures who do powerful stuff. Good compost is like good qualitative research. It needs planning, careful attention and the right mix of ingredients to grow healthy, productive and useful results.

A rigorous qualitative researcher does not ignore the critical moments, sanitize them or dress them up behind closed doors. This is what our authors demonstrate in their negotiations with the research process. Good qualitative research includes critical moments, struggles, resistances, pleasure and a personal journey. These ingredients add rigour to our work. Rigorous qualitative research negotiates the structures that constrain us from speaking, helping to blur the rigid boundaries between life and research. Attending to the detail, the relationships, the ethics, the conventions and structures, is also being rigorous. Certain research practices will always confront us. However, as many of the writers in this collection demonstrate, negotiating them is important in the development of competent and rigorous researchers. They stepped around the wall of silence that surrounds subjective experiences, radical processes and messy moments, and said, 'This is what happened, this is how I negotiated it, and this is what I now know'. Rigour, then, in qualitative research, is just as rigorous as in quantitative research, but we retain within this concept and practice the complexity of context and the personal voices that epitomize qualitative research.

Reframing

Throughout each of the five themes explored above and across the various authors' experiences runs a collective theme: reframing. We have reframed a number of old debates (such as the qualitative/quantitative divide, rigour and subjectivity), creating a new context of inclusiveness, personal validity and multiple realities. We have taken research out of the traditional individual researcher's 'black box' of trouble-free research with set methodologies, and we have presented research that rejoices in collectives, blurred boundaries and the real lived experiences of the researchers. We have explored the dynamics of self and of knowledge, in the fluidity of evolution that is research. Reframing allows the researcher to turn problems into opportunities and restrictions into liberation.

Concluding . . .

Researching is a social practice shaped by the discursive field of our age and culture, which, as demonstrated in a number of the chapters, is still largely informed by the dominance of scientific and economic rationality. The hegemony of these discourses can blind us to what else is present. Our purpose in writing this book has been to demonstrate that qualitative research is an ordinary activity as well as an illuminating one. It is not separate from our daily lives and relationships. However, this fact is often disguised. We have shown that it is nonetheless present. In making people's *already existing* research strategies visible, i.e. the authors were asked to reveal their critical moments, we have opened the space for conversation and learning. Each of the knowledge(s) that have been produced is partial, never complete, leaving the space open for you as the reader to add your local knowledge. Now, we want to leave these stories to speak for themselves . . .

References

Foucault, M. (1980) 'Truth and power'. In *Power/Knowledge: Selected Interviews and Writings by Michel Foucault* (C. Gordon, ed.), pp. 109–133. Brighton: Harvester Press.

Grumet, M. (1990) 'Show and tell: a response to the value issues in alternative paradigms for inquiry'. In *The Paradigm Dialogue* (E. Guba and Y. Lincoln, eds), pp. 333–342. Newbury Park: Sage.

van Gennep, A. (1960) *The Rite of Passage*. Chicago: Chicago University Press.

Section Two

Lost in time and space

2

The fractured lens: methodology in perspective

Heather D'Cruz

Qualitative researchers are faced with a proliferation of methodologies and methods that often clash. The mainstream story is that:

- one cannot mix methodologies or use conflicting ones
- the methodology is separate from the research and researcher
- one has one's methodology clearly defined before embarking on the research
- the research fits the methodology – a linear process.

These rules can sometimes lead to confusion and paralysis, and do not fully reflect the process researchers go through as they negotiate the literature. Alternative perspectives (e.g. Stanley and Wise, 1993; Bryman and Burgess, 1994; Denzin and Lincoln, 1994) challenge the mainstream research story of one methodology and linear, sanitized processes. The purpose of this chapter is to extend these critiques by placing methodology in (practical) perspective of my PhD project. A metaphor of a *fractured lens* represents my alternative to the mainstream story.

I discuss the methodological and ethical issues associated with a fractured lens, particularly that of researcher objectivity/subjectivity, and the relationship between *researcher* and *researched*. I then reconstruct the process by which I composed my fractured lens, telling the tale from the vantage point of the 'present' time and place. I conclude by reflecting on how fractured lenses place methodology in perspective.

Background

This story of my fractured lens operates at two levels: as how I constructed a way of understanding my PhD project, and as a narrative of methodology in (practical) perspective.

My PhD topic, 'Constructing meanings and identities in practice: Child protection in Western Australia' (D'Cruz, 1999), analyses how the diverse events reported to child protection organizations are given official meaning as 'maltreatment' of particular 'types'; and how the identities of 'child', 'parent' and 'person believed responsible' are also constructed, rather than taken-for-granted, categories.

The processes of construction are told from the perspectives of child protection workers, represented in case files (documents), narratives (semi-structured interviews) and situated interactions (participant observation). Individual practices are contextualized within child protection policies as discourses (Bacchi, 1998), and as situated in place (practice sites and cultures) and time.

Place and time are also important for contextualizing the project and the construction of my fractured lens. Whilst I am registered for the PhD at the Department of Applied Social Science, Lancaster University, UK, the research is about child protection practice in Western Australia. Thus, place is important for understanding any reference to particular locations as central to the telling of the tale and to distance, bridged by email and phone calls, and occasional visits to the University.

Part-time is more than a descriptive category of registration and time commitment to the project. Time contextualizes the unfolding of this story over several lived years, yet the actual PhD time cannot be measured in this way. 'Why are you taking so long?' is a frequent question, more often from people who have never done PhDs or whose experiences have differed considerably, in terms of paid time and other supports. However, to mix one's metaphors, the 'loneliness of the long distance researcher' was/is a key feature in the construction of a fractured lens, as there was/is time to reflect upon the nexus between theories and applications and to try out different lenses. A single lens could well have been a consequence of more constrained time frames, such as four years for full time (and funded) students.

Philosophical and intellectual assumptions

Ontological and epistemological assumptions are integral to and inform methodology (Stanley and Wise, 1990, 1993; Guba and Lincoln, 1994). They include the conceptualization, design, implementation and analysis of the project. Methodology, as defined by Stanley and Wise (1990, p. 26), 'is a "perspective" or very broad theoretically informed framework ... which may or may not specify its own particular "appropriate" research method/s or technique/s'. Epistemology as a 'theory of knowledge' would thus inform methodology, through considerations of the nature of knowledge and how it can be known and validated, and what the relationship should be between 'knowing [i.e. epistemology] and being [i.e. ontology]' (Stanley and Wise, 1990, p. 26).

The epistemological assumptions for my project are that knowledge is socially constructed, and that there is no value-free science (Stanley and Wise, 1990). This constructionist perspective challenges the positivist dichotomy between 'research object' and 'research subject', and the consequent positioning between the researched (as passive objects) and the researcher (as one who sees and knows). Ontological assumptions are of complex layers and fault lines of reality, not of a single coherent object to be discovered (Stanley and Wise, 1990).

The fractured lens is a metaphor for methodology: 'ways of knowing' as 'ways of seeing' (Haraway, 1991). Technology extends the mind's eye: that of the seer and the effects on how and what is seen.

The fractured lens: objectivity and subjectivity, objects and subjects

The metaphor of a fractured lens poses methodological and ethical considerations, particularly of researcher objectivity and subjectivity, and the relationship between researcher and researched.

An actual lens, as a technology of seeing, places a distance and perceptual frame between the researcher as seer and the researched as seen (Haraway, 1991). It suggests that the researcher is objective, being distanced from what is being researched. Yet the material technology of seeing influences and circumscribes the perceptual field, so that what is seen is as much a feature of how it is seen. Thus, physiological perception enhanced and influenced by material technology may be extended as an analogy for the way in which a metaphoric lens as an epistemological position may also challenge the apparent objectivity of the researcher.

Instead, the epistemological positioning of the researcher operates as an intellectual (and perceptual/cognitive) technology of seeing (and doing) the entire research project. This includes the way in which the literature is read, the selection of the research question, the design and analysis, and the eventual writing up (Stanley and Wise, 1993).

Epistemological positioning is integral to researcher history and biography, personal values, beliefs and identities. 'Subjectivity matters' (Riessman, 1994) in the conceptualization, design, analysis and reporting of research (Stanley and Wise, 1993).

In my case, as a 'positioned investigator' (Riessman, 1994), my interest in how social categories such as gender, class, race/ethnicity, sexual preference and disability intersect in the practical constructions of meanings, identities and their implications, is influenced by my personal biography and history and reflections on my interactions with others. Thus for me it is impossible to claim objectivity as a researcher, when my personal engagement is so interwoven with the intellectual and political aspects of the project (Denzin and Lincoln, 1994).

The other key methodological and ethical issue arises from the way in which a fractured lens may constitute the relationship between researcher and researched, as subjects and objects. Traditionally, the researched are constituted as objects of knowledge, who may be known by the researcher as knowledge expert (Stanley and Wise, 1993). A lens has the potential to operate in ways that entrench this duality and inequality in the relationship. A real lens, for example in a microscope or a camera, places and organizes the objects of interest within the perceptual field of the seer. A methodological lens may do the same thing unless the researcher actively promotes an egalitarian relationship.

In my case, I extended the metaphor of the fractured lens by naming the type of lens it might be, and therefore its part in constituting the research relationship. For example, had my lens been a microscope, greater distancing would be suggested, with potential for the object/subject separation to be maintained. The image of the research relationship and associated identities would be of a large, powerful researcher, and small, powerless researched. It would also constitute the researcher primarily as the detached observer of the researched and their interactive contexts.

Instead, my lens was a pair of glasses which I as researcher could wear as I participated within and observed the context with the researched as equal participants. These glasses could operate as binoculars if I wished to see the bigger picture of interactions and patterns from the top of the hill. They could also operate as ordinary glasses within the context of daily interactions in which I participated.

Constructing my fractured lens

In this section I tell the tale of how I constructed my fractured lens, from the perspective of 'the present' (i.e. August 1998). The representation of this process is therefore a relatively tidy (and linear) version of an iterative (and messy) process. However, I have structured this story by different devices: a description of the selection of each piece of the lens, interspersed with a reflexive analysis of the critique of its adequacy and the subsequent casting about/selection of yet another piece. This reflexive analysis is presented in italics to differentiate it from the descriptive and perhaps more overt process. I have also structured this narrative as a linear chronological process in which time, place and stage of the project were highly relevant in the construction of the fractured lens.

January 1993

My introduction to 'postmodernism: the theory' occurred literally on day one, when my then supervisor gave me a book by Boyne and Rattansi (1990), *Postmodernism and Society*. Although the topic stated in my application was 'the social construction of child abuse', more academic sociology was a foreign land to me as a policy officer/researcher in the Western Australian public service. I had never heard of postmodernism, and this particular text talked a lot about culture, art and architecture.

What has this to do with child protection? (panic-stricken) Am I going to be able to do this thing called a PhD? I don't understand what these people are talking about. You have to be really intelligent to get a PhD. Will I make it?

I spoke of these concerns, was pronounced 'atheoretical', and given a range of basic texts (which discussed both postmodernism and poststructuralism – extremely confusing for a novice!). These texts were more relevant, although still somewhat inaccessible, mainly because of the different language (vocabulary and its presentation). However, I persevered and a whole new world opened up to me. Concepts of difference, the explosion of categories, and power as relations of practice were especially important, as they started to give some pointers for the project, its purpose and its design.

By the end of 1993, Foucault in particular emerged as a primary source of theory. His concept of discourse (power/knowledge) was a new way of seeing the articulation of professional knowledge and professional legitimacy (as power) (Foucault, 1972, 1977, 1980, 1983). His 'genealogical method' (Foucault, 1965, 1978) showed the shifting meaning of 'protection' in relation to children and parents in Western Australia, from colonization to contemporary times, within related institutional contexts. Language is central to the representation of meanings and identities, not as a one-to-one correspondence, but as constructing particular images of reality (Foucault, 1983). The body of the individual is a site of power/knowledge (Hewitt, 1991); professional practices of surveillance and normalization operate to discipline individuals ('bio-power') and populations ('bio-politics') simultaneously, and to know them respectively as 'cases' and as 'statistics' (Hacking, 1990).

These concepts facilitated understanding child protection as discourse, constituted in institutional and professional power/knowledge relations over time and place (Hacking, 1991). Individual bodies (children, parents and 'persons believed responsible') operate as sites of power/knowledge, whereby professionals simultaneously examine and divide 'abnormal' from 'normal' identities: as 'maltreated' (or not), as 'responsible' (or not), as 'unprotective' (or not). Children and families who are reported to child protection organizations on the ground that 'something happened' to the child become 'cases' which must be investigated by child protection practitioners. The outcomes of these investigative processes are represented as statistical categories, named as 'maltreatment' of various 'types', and the child acquires an identity of 'victim' in relation to someone identified as 'person believed responsible'. All these categories are official ways of naming the purpose of child protection intervention in relation to problematic relationships between a child-as-victim and a person who is responsible. The categories also represent official and legitimate knowledge of the 'true' boundaries and dimensions of child protection as a political and professional activity (Eckenrode *et al.*, 1988; Finkelhor *et al.*, 1990; Winefield and Bradley, 1992; Ards and Harrell, 1993; Finkelhor, 1994; Bertolli *et al.*, 1995).

Foucault thus formed my first lens (and at the time, I believed, was 'the methodological approach').

However, whilst Foucault provided these excellent ways of seeing the more macroformulations of meanings and identities, categorized as child, parent and protection, I felt uneasy that I could only image his concepts as 'big pictures' and aerial maps of the discursive territory. My initial unease was primarily an intuitive reaction, which I later formulated as questions and issues.

Can I make the leap from Foucault's concepts to looking at micropractices, when I have no specific concepts from Foucault to justify or name these processes? I can't see how Foucault's concepts and methods help me to understand the social practices that contribute to the bigger picture. I probably don't really understand Foucault all that well.

I was much relieved to find that Dreyfus and Rabinow (1982), as Foucauldian scholars, provided insights into my uneasy formulations.

I sought an approach which would connect with Foucault, in particular his concepts of power/knowledge, understandings of 'the body' and identity, and language as central to discourse. These criteria influenced my search for another piece of my theoretical lens.

1994

'Miraculous' is the way I described my discovery of Bourdieu's 'theory of practice'. However, the miraculous usually has some practical grounding. In my case, my heightened consciousness of what was needed intersected with my immersion in various texts on ethnomethodology, sociolinguistic theories and analysis, and, most importantly, voluntary attendance at a subject, Language, Ideology and Power, taught at Lancaster University by Norman Fairclough (Department of Linguistics) and Mick Dillon (Department of Politics). This subject included Bourdieu's work for its contribution to understanding language as power relations. I was fascinated by the way in which language could be analysed as a critique of institutional and social relations and power. However, it was not entirely clear at the time exactly how this might be relevant to my project.

Bourdieu's (1990, 1991) theory of practice, grounded in anthropological studies, bridged the conceptual gap between Foucault's analyses of knowledge embedded in institutional power relations, and social relations. Child protection discourse (as capital) could be produced as particular social practices between particular identities representing professionals, parents and children. These practices relied on linguistic transactions, embedded in relations of power. Differential power of participants as 'linguistic capital' was associated with differential value given to the capital each possessed in terms of social, economic, cultural and symbolic dimensions.

'You can't use Foucault and Bourdieu together. They are epistemologically different' (female academic sociologist). Panic-stricken, I consulted my supervisor, Dr Sue Wise, who said, 'You are not a sociologist, but an applied social researcher. You can use any approaches you like if they will help your project'. This statement was encouraging and liberating, as it affirmed my diffident audacity in critiquing these theoretical approaches and scholars.

1995

I was still employed by the Western Australian public service as a research officer in a child protection/welfare organization, so was viewing that world through a pair of lenses: one that was my fractured constructionism, and the other the clear, unitary lens of the 'bureau-professional' (Dingwall et al., 1983). This made the daily view of my work somewhat uncomfortable, but I adapted to its disorienting effects.

However, I again became uneasy; this time about the ethics of a constructionist perspective, particularly in relation to a socially problematic issue, child maltreatment. The scholarly literature critiques the 'epistemological and ethical relativism' (Smart, 1993) associated with constructionism: the descent into scepticism (Rosenau, 1992), its potential for extreme individualism, and the destruction of political solidarity (Bauman, 1991, 1993). Having practised as a social worker and a policy officer in this child protection/welfare organization I had seen children with injuries, and there was plenty of public and professional knowledge about the tragedies involving children in the care of parents and other caregivers (Parton, 1985, 1991; Johnson, 1990; Wise, 1990; Armytage and Reeves, 1992). I was also conscious of my intellectualizing about the problem, bordering on dismissal of the very real daily concerns of my social work colleagues and, more importantly, the lived experiences of children.

I was loath to give up my new-found perspective, which was intellectually exciting and challenging, but ethically controversial. I then recollected reading an article by Heap on constructionism, in which he discussed these issues as 'monist' and 'dualist' intellectual positions.

Heap (1995) differentiated between monist positions, which see all reality as constructions, and dualist positions, which see that reality has some material basis, but is given meaning through constructions by participants. Therefore, I positioned myself as a dualist, which meant I could continue to see (and know) through both fractured and unitary lenses and could also accommodate ethics, thereby reconnecting 'intellect' with 'emotion' (Stanley and Wise, 1993).

And there, I thought, I have resolved it!

The next issue to be confronted was how to analyse my data. Local experts in Western Australia insisted that 'grounded theory' (Glaser and Straus, 1967; Straus and Corbin, 1990, 1994) was the approach. Grounded theory assumes that the researcher's theoretical perspective is not imposed on the researched, but allows the theory to emerge 'inductively' through 'interplay with data ... throughout the course of a research project' (Straus and Corbin, 1994, p. 274). By appropriate analytical methods, in particular 'coding' and the 'constant comparative method', core and axial theoretical concepts emerge.

I was uncomfortable with the approach because I could not see how theory could emerge independently of the researcher (Bryman, 1988; Stanley and Wise, 1990; Bryman and Burgess, 1994; Denzin, 1994; Denzin and Lincoln, 1994), especially as I was influenced by the assumption of the researcher's 'positioned subjectivity' (Riessman, 1994). However, my idiosyncratic way of seeing and doing probably exercised the greatest influence on my eventual rejection of this analytical method.

Through immersion in my data, I had already commenced an analytical process that did not fit comfortably with this one. 'How do these codes and categories necessarily tell me about how the workers construct what happened to the child as a category of maltreatment, and who was responsible? How does this approach help me to understand how child and parent are constructed as identities? There's too much detail, it's taking ages to do the coding, it's too structured, there are too many sequential stages ... What am I meant to do next? I can see themes emerging without doing this process. How do I deal with large chunks of text and how can I link the codes and categories to a context? Am I coding words or sentences or paragraphs or whole chunks of text that relate to a specific question or issue? Should I use respondents' languages represented in the texts as my codes, or should I use the language of my theoretical perspective? How do I look at these different languages representing ways of seeing that are different from mine? How does having my own fractured lens relate to this?'

1996

The 'dualist' position (e.g. Heap, 1995) is considered to be inconsistent with a constructionist perspective, as it perpetuates the positivist distinction between object and subject (Guba and Lincoln, 1994).

'Here we go again!'

By this time, I was able to enhance my understanding of the ethical contradictions presented by a constructionist position and the adoption of the dualist position discussed by Heap (1995). The discussion of realism and relativism by Edwards *et al.* (1995) helped me to differentiate between the real as the actual experiences of children, and how these experiences might be manifested materially in their bodies, as injuries and even more extremely as death. However, the relativism associated with constructionism pertained to the meanings given by different people, including the child, the parent, the person believed responsible and the child protection worker, to these material experiences. This dualist viewpoint was eminently feasible for my project's ethical position.

'What am I going to do about my data analysis? How does Bourdieu's concept of linguistic capital as the currency of social transactions embedded in power actually get played out? Is it enough to make claims from the data about how the processes of construction happen? Do I need a method (as a systematic "how to do") which justifies the analytical process and therefore validates the claims I am making?'

In July 1996, my move into full-time academia coincided with my discovery that I was now seeing through two fractured lenses, rather than the combination of fractured and whole when I started this project.

1997

Whilst on my annual visit to Lancaster University, I was browsing in an Edinburgh bookshop and again my miracle happened. I discovered Potter's (1996) *Representing Reality: Discourse, Rhetoric and Social Construction*, which brought together the analytical methods discussed in various texts on sociolinguistics and ethnomethodology (Pithouse, 1987; Antaki, 1988; Smith, 1990) within the social constructionist perspective. Potter focuses on how rhetorical devices organize the factual status of descriptions. Rhetorical devices are a range of linguistic resources and techniques by which practical fact construction (as 'reification') or fact destruction (as 'ironization') occurs (Potter, 1996, p. 121). Through rhetorical devices, linguistic practices of particular participants become devices of power in producing legitimate knowledge as discourse, and de-legitimating other versions. Discourse analysis extends ethnographic understandings to *how* accounts are 'established as literal and objective, and what it is being used to do' (Potter, 1996, pp. 105–106).

Putting the pieces together

Potter (1996, p. 105) reworks 'discourse' as:

> the concern ... with talk and texts as parts of social practices. *This is a somewhat broader than the conversation analytic concern with talk-in-interaction, but rather more focused on the specifics of people's practices than the Foucauldian notion of a discourse as a set of statements that formulate objects and subjects. (original emphasis)*

My reading of Potter is that it is possible to connect both Foucault and Bourdieu by the linkage of abstract 'texts' and 'sets of statements' with 'social (and linguistic) practices'. 'Linguistic construction' is a theme in post-structuralism, including Foucault's work on discourse (Potter, 1996), and in ethnomethodology, which focuses on the indexicality, reflexivity and situatedness of people's practices through language (Potter, 1996).

However, discourses are not 'unlocated universes of meaning' (Rodger, 1991, p. 68). Instead, the deployment of rhetorical devices in the practical construction of meanings and identities must be located within cultural, structural and discursive contexts of identity; for example, a mother's practices in relation to her child are embedded and understood within the 'cultural idealization of mothering' (Rose, 1989), not solely as a specific and situated incident. Capital associated with particular identities as 'sites of power' (Barrett, 1987) is differentially allocated (Bourdieu, 1990, 1991), along with the distribution of opportunities to deploy rhetorical devices; for example, the processes of exclusion of 'abnormals' or 'deviants' from construction of legitimate accounts (Smith, 1990). The privileging of particular constructions over others is also not just a feature of rhetorical techniques (as power neutral), but is contingent on the relations of power by which different versions are validated or not, depending on the identities and positionings of participants (Barrett, 1987).

1998

By June I had sent my supervisor two draft chapters, analysing the practical constructions of how a report that 'something happened' to a child was given discursive meaning as a 'type of maltreatment'; and how a discursive identity, 'person believed responsible', was associated with a particular 'someone'. I had commenced writing my final analytical chapter, Constructing the 'child', the 'parent' and 'protection'. The complexity of the analytical process looking through my fractured lens was cause for panic and doubt, as exemplified in this email message from me to my supervisor.

(The message is quoted verbatim, although with emphasis added, with only text irrelevant to this discussion deleted.)

From: Heather D'Cruz
Sent: Monday, 15 June 1998 12:43
To: S.Wise @ XXX
Subject: thesis

Sue

[...] My proposed chapter linking Foucault, Bourdieu and Potter in the section before the analysis of cases commences discuss[es] the relevant concepts and what they mean etc.... [...] F. as himself is 'useful' for the lit. review and genealogy and therefore I can deal with him and then get into those chapters – and then ... I will have to launch into why B. and P. and their connections to F. and how these three operate together in different combinations in the analysis of cases.
Another issue arising – I don't necessarily use Potter all the time and esp. in the last chapter on child, parent and protection – it seems to go back more to the discursive and F. in practice (less to do with contests about who is who

and what is what as per Potter, more to do with how these identities are discursively constructed [assumptions] and how this is represented in the worker's texts). Not quite clear why this is – a failing of the approach? There is some Potter, but not very much as not all that helpful. He was more so in the other two analysis chapters.

Is this complicating it all too much – my greatest anxiety is the examiners saying 'fail' because it is too complicated – why didn't you use just one approach etc. *I suppose the answer is partly related to data sources and partly to what is emerging and therefore needing to be shown. Is this a passable answer – Also an issue of 'how is it grounded' if I am reading it in particular ways? (methodological issue about grounded approaches I suppose).[. . .].*

This email message shows how insidious is the myth of the single lens, as I had not been aware of what I had written, until I reread it some weeks later.

My supervisor's reply challenged the myth of single lens, and encouraged the alternative of a fractured lens, as reflective of social research in practice.

From: wise s [SMTP:s.wise@XXX]
Sent: Monday, 15 June 1998 22:30
To: Heather D'Cruz
Subject: Thesis

[. . .] I don't think it matters that you use more of Potter in one analysis chapter and more of Foucault in another – you've set out your stall as using helpful analytic tools from each, so I don't think you need to worry about using each of them 'equally'. In any case, it can be a legitimate part of your discussion about why some aspects of the theoretical work are more useful in the actual analysis than others. [. . .].

The fractured lens: methodology in perspective

In this chapter, I have put 'methodology in (practical) perspective' through the metaphor of a fractured lens, as a way of seeing, knowing (and doing) my PhD research. I have also discussed the epistemological, methodological and ethical issues associated with a fractured lens, and how epistemology and methodology cannot be separated from ethics. For my project, my fractured lens, which juxtaposes primarily Foucault, Bourdieu and Potter, helps me to see how reports that someone did something to a child are transformed by practical constructions into official meanings, such as 'types of maltreatment', 'protection', identities of 'person believed responsible', 'child' and 'parent'.

Thus a fractured lens has put my methodology in perspective by showing why and how multiple ways of seeing were and are necessary for my project, making explicit both the academic analysis as the public and sanitized version of social research, and the generally invisible, private and messy processes, fears and challenges behind it. A fractured lens allows for multiple, if somewhat disjointed, ways of seeing a fractured reality which can be known in different ways, yet can be connected, if somewhat tenuously at times.

Yet this chapter is not intended to represent a firm conclusion, somehow proving that single lens methodology is wrong and that a fractured lens is right, thus re-polarizing the debate. Instead, this particular narrative of methodology in (practical) perspective is intended to open up, rather than close off, the possibilities for seeing and knowing.

As I sit now, writing this story, my fractured lens may be best represented as a pair of very odd glasses, with both lenses fractured. It presents two observations for ongoing reflection in/on research practice. One is that I have not been able to maintain the initial rather uncomfortable fractured/unitary binocular lenses, instead having to fracture both lenses. The second observation is that the multiple fragments still had to be combined as a single lens, to produce some kind of wholeness and coherence. The challenge for us as researchers is how to allow for multiple ways of seeing, whether through single or fractured lenses, instead of debates about false dichotomies and hierarchies of knowledge and knowing.

References

Antaki, C. (ed.) (1988) *Analysing Everyday Explanation: A Casebook of Methods*. London: Sage.

Ards, S. and Harrell, A. (1993) Reporting of child maltreatment: a secondary analysis of the national incidence surveys. *Child Abuse and Neglect*, **17**(3), 337–344.

Armytage, P. and Reeves, C. (1992). Practice insights as revealed by child death inquiries in Victoria and overseas. In *The Practice of Child Protection: Australian Approaches* (G. Calvert, A. Ford and P. Parkinson, eds), pp. 122–140. Sydney: Hale and Iremonger.

Bacchi, C. (1998). Policy as discourse: What does it mean? Where does it get us? Paper presented to the Postmodernism in Practice Conference: The Discursive Construction of Knowledge Group, 25 February–1 March, University of Adelaide, South Australia.

Barrett, M. (1987) The concept of difference. *Feminist Review*, **26**, 29–41.

Bauman, Z. (1991) *Postmodernity: Chance or Menace*. Lancaster: Centre for the Study of Cultural Values, Lancaster University, UK.

Bauman, Z. (1993) *Postmodern Ethics*. Oxford: Blackwell.

Bertolli, J., Morgenstern, H. and Sorenson, S. B. (1995) Estimating the occurrence of child maltreatment and risk-factor effects: benefits of a mixed-design strategy in epidemiologic research. *Child Abuse and Neglect*, **19**(8), 1007–1016.

Bourdieu, P. (1990) *The Logic of Practice* (R. Nice, trans.). Cambridge: Polity Press.

Bourdieu, P. (1991) *Language and Symbolic Power* (G. Raymond and M. Adamson, trans.). Cambridge: Polity Press.

Boyne, R. and Rattansi, A. (eds) (1990) *Postmodernism and Society*. London: Macmillan.

Bryman, A. (1988) *Quantity and Quality in Social Research*. London: Routledge.

Bryman, A. and Burgess, R. (eds) (1994) *Analyzing Qualitative Data*. London: Routledge.

D'Cruz, H. (1999) Constructing meanings and identities in practice: Child protection in Western Australia. PhD thesis, Department of Applied Social Science, Lancaster University, UK.

Denzin, N. K. (1994) The art and politics of interpretation. In *Handbook of Qualitative Research* (N. K. Denzin and Y. S. Lincoln, eds), pp. 500–515. Thousand Oaks: Sage.

Denzin, N. K. and Lincoln, Y. S. (1994) Strategies of inquiry. In *Handbook of Qualitative Research* (N. K. Denzin and Y. S. Lincoln, eds), pp. 199–208. Thousand Oaks: Sage.

Dingwall, R., Eekelaar, J. and Murray, T. (1983) *The Protection of Children: State Intervention in Family Life*. Oxford: Basil Blackwell.

Dreyfus, H. L. and Rabinow, P. (1982) *Michel Foucault: Beyond Structuralism and Hermeneutics*. Hemel Hempstead: Harvester Wheatsheaf.

Eckenrode, J., Powers, J., Doris, J., Munsch, J. and Bolger, N. (1988) Substantiation of child abuse and neglect reports. *Journal of Consulting and Clinical Psychology*, **56**(1), 9–16.

Edwards, D., Ashmore, M. and Potter, J. (1995). Death and furniture: the rhetoric, politics and theology of bottom line arguments against relativism. *History of the Human Sciences*, **8**, 25–49.

Finkelhor, D. (1994) The international epidemiology of child sexual abuse. *Child Abuse and Neglect*, **18**(5), 409–418.

Finkelhor, D., Hotaling, G., Lewis, I. A. and Smith, C. (1990). Sexual abuse in a national survey of adult men and women: Prevalence, characteristics, and risk factors. *Child Abuse and Neglect*, **14**(1), 19–28.

Foucault, M. (1965) *Madness and Civilization: A History of Insanity in the Age of Reason* (R. Howard, trans.). London: Routledge.

Foucault, M. (1972) *The Archaeology of Knowledge* (A. Sheridan, trans.). London: Tavistock.

Foucault, M. (1977) *Discipline and Punish: The Birth of the Prison* (A. Sheridan, trans.). London: Penguin.

Foucault, M. (1978) *The History of Sexuality: An Introduction*, Vol. 1 (R. Hurley, trans.). Cambridge: Penguin.

Foucault, M. (1980) *Power/Knowledge: Selected Interviews and Other Writings, 1972–1977* (C. Gordon, ed.). Hemel Hempstead: The Harvester Press.

Foucault, M. (1983) *This Is Not a Pipe* (J. Harkness, trans. and ed.). Berkeley and Los Angeles: University of California Press.

Glaser, B. and Straus, A. (1967) *The Discovery of Grounded Theory*. Chicago: Aldine.

Guba, E. and Lincoln, Y. (1994) Competing paradigms in qualitative research. In *Handbook of Qualitative Research* (N. K. Denzin and Y. S. Lincoln, eds), pp. 105–117). Thousand Oaks: Sage.

Hacking, I. (1990) *The Taming of Chance*. Cambridge: Cambridge University Press.

Hacking, I. (1991) The making and molding of child abuse. *Critical Inquiry*, **17**, 253–288.

Haraway, D. (1991) *Simians, Cyborgs and Women*. London: Free Association Books.

Heap, J. L. (1995) Constructionism in the rhetoric and practice of fourth generation evaluation. *Evaluation and Program Planning*, **18**(1), 51–61.

Hewitt, M. (1991) Bio-politics and social policy: Foucault's account of welfare. In *The Body: Social Process and Cultural Theory* (M. Featherstone, M. Hepworth and B. Turner, eds), pp. 225–255. London: Sage.

Johnson, J. (1990) *What Lisa Knew: The Truth and Lies of the Steinberg Case*. London: Bloomsbury.

Parton, N. (1985) *The Politics of Child Abuse*. London: Macmillan.

Parton, N. (1991) *Governing the Family: Child Care, Child Protection and the State*. London: Macmillan.

Pithouse, A. (1987) *Social Work: The Social Organisation of an Invisible Trade*. Aldershot: Avebury.

Potter, J. (1996) *Representing Reality: Discourse, Rhetoric and Social Construction*. London: Sage.

Riessman, C. K. (ed.) (1994) *Qualitative Studies in Social Work Research*. Thousand Oaks: Sage.

Rodger, J. (1991) Discourse analysis and social relationships in social work. *British Journal of Social Work*, **21**, 63–79.

Rose, N. (1989) *Governing the Soul: The Shaping of the Private Self*. London: Routledge.

Rosenau, P. (1992) *Post-modernism and the Social Sciences: Insights, Inroads and Intrusions*. Princeton: Princeton University Press.

Smart, B. (1993) *Postmodernity*. London: Routledge.

Smith, D. (1990) K is mentally ill. In *Texts, Facts and Femininity: Exploring the Relations of Ruling* (D. Smith, ed.), pp. 12–52. London: Routledge.

Stanley, L. and Wise, S. (1990) Method, methodology and epistemology in feminist research processes. In *Feminist Praxis: Research, Theory and Epistemology in Feminist Sociology* (L. Stanley, ed.), pp. 20–60. London: Routledge.

Stanley, L. and Wise, S. (1993) *Breaking Out Again: Feminist Ontology and Epistemology*. London: Routledge.

Straus, A. and Corbin, J. (1990) *Basics of Qualitative Research: Grounded Theory Procedures and Techniques.* Newbury Park: Sage.

Straus, A. and Corbin, J. (1994) Grounded theory methodology: an overview. In *Handbook of Qualitative Research* (N. K. Denzin and Y. S. Lincoln, eds), pp. 273–285. Thousand Oaks: Sage.

Winefield, H. R. and Bradley, P. W. (1992) Substantiation of reported child abuse or neglect: predictors and implications. *Child Abuse and Neglect*, **16**(5), pp. 661–672.

Wise, S. (1990) Becoming a feminist social worker. In *Feminist Praxis* (L. Stanley, ed.), pp. 236–249. London: Routledge.

3

Being a methodological space cadet

Charles Higgs and Lindy McAllister

Structure

This chapter takes the form of a dialogue between a novice [N] methodological space cadet (Charles) and a more experienced [E] methodological space cadet (Lindy). Charles is at the beginning of his doctoral studies; Lindy is writing up her doctoral thesis. For both Lindy and Charles, their doctoral research projects have been their first venture into the unknown world of qualitative research. Lindy has since undertaken other qualitative research projects with Masters students. A third dimension to this chapter has been added to the work, that of a reflective commentary on the dialogue, written by both authors. The voices of the novice and experienced methodological space cadet are indicated by [N] and [E] respectively, and the reflective commentary appears as plain text. The dialogue was conducted by email over a number of months, and the commentary was written as the work progressed and also as a reflective process. As a document it reflects the questions, thoughts and ideas that were generated throughout the dialogue, but by its very nature it cannot fully encapsulate the angst, frustration, wonder and excitement that lie between the lines. Our story begins with Charles' reflections on the start of his journey.

N: I recently attended a university workshop where new Research Masters and PhD students were discussing the events of the initial months of their respective courses. As they spoke I heard my own words of a year ago echoing in my mind. The concerns and issues that they raised, particularly regarding methodologies, were issues that I had raised with my supervisor and colleagues at the beginning of my doctoral journey.

The conversations that occurred at the beginning of my research journey have influenced the structure of this chapter. The chapter covers the following themes:

- Lift-off (the journey begins)
- Lost in space
- Signposts and speed limits?
- Splashdown!

What is a space cadet?

N: The term 'space cadet' is a nebulous term referring to anyone venturing into some form of the unknown, and as a novice researcher I saw myself as a type of 'space cadet', venturing into the relatively unexplored realms of my own research. There was a certain excitement at the beginning of my journey that in hindsight overshadowed the apprehension and confusion lurking in the corners of my mind.

The origin of the 'space cadet' concept lies in a 1950s black and white TV series called *Tom Corbett, Space Cadet*. It was an innovative and exploratory series that set the standards for science fiction series in the years to come:

> Early science fiction television shows were part of the 'cutting' edge of technology for the 1950s with live broadcasts & special effects. The 1950s 'new media' (television) was changing from the 'horse opera' of the past to the 'space opera' of the future. (Pippen, 1998, p. 1)

Lift-off (the journey begins)

N: Like the TV series space cadet, I wanted my thesis to be futuristic and cutting edge, without fully comprehending what that meant. I wanted to be creative and tell my 'story', however that unfolded.

A thesis can be seen as a type of personal story, as is articulated here by Mills (1994, pp. 2–3):

> Your thesis is a creative story. Your story. The story of your research or, for the most part, your re-search. And, in generic terms, your thesis belongs to the category of the epic. A thesis is an epic. We have come to associate the word epic with an exceptionally long story or endeavour of some kind. But, strictly speaking, it refers to that genre which describes a journey, specifically a journey in search of one's identity as with, for example, Ulysses. Viewed from this perspective, your thesis is your journey of search, re-search, for an identity.

N: I wanted my journey to be one involving myself and others. I had had some exposure to quantitative research, but it lacked the 'me' component I felt should be included in my research. When I heard about qualitative research, I thought that this was the type of research that I wanted to do. But wasn't research fundamentally about statistics, double-blind tests, and the like?

E: It is not uncommon for people to view research as being based only in the positivist paradigm. My experience was that I was 'raised' in a positivist paradigm and had done research quite happily in that mode, because the sorts of questions that I was asking were best answered in that paradigm. But when I started my thesis (McAllister, 2001), I was drawn to a question that could best be answered in the interpretive paradigm. It took me some time to discover that it existed. Once I did, I still had no idea of what methodologies I would use. I finally came to storying because it provided the best fit. I guess I was sympathetic to interpretive research because of my recreational reading of ethno-graphies.

Traditionally research was viewed as the domain of technical rationality and scientific order, but now the boundaries of research are expanding to include areas previously unheard of:

> . . . where only statistics and experimental designs, and survey research once stood, researchers have opened up to ethnography, unstructured interviewing, textual analysis, and historical studies. Where "We're doing science" was once the watchword, scholars are now experimenting with the boundaries of interpretation. (Denzin and Lincoln, 1994, p. ix)

A lifetime of training and conditioning

Positivism, with its pursuit of unique answers to finite questions, dominates the compulsory school years. During these formative years we are encour-aged to believe that the 'hard sciences' are of greater value than the 'soft sciences', and that order and objectivity are desirable; chaos and subjectivity are incompatible with sound research.

This positivist view of the world often continues into post-secondary education, and although some are fortunate enough to gain exposure to alternate philosophies during their undergraduate years, the positivist (and predominantly masculine) world view impacts upon many people's approach to research. Positivist research aims to 'measure, test hypotheses, discover, predict, explain, control, generalize, identify cause–effect relation-ship' (Higgs, 1998, p. 146).

The imposition of linear thought processing and the dominant positivist paradigm on our decisions regarding research methodology is indicative of the emphasis placed on the search for measurement and answers over the desire to interpret and understand. This imposition can be external, for example from a procedural perspective (our supervisors, research review committee), or it can be internal, in the form of our epistemology and how it was influenced during our formative years.

N: This is the situation I found myself in. My undergraduate training was strongly grounded in the positivist paradigm. Even before this my Higher School Certificate subjects included maths, physics and chemistry, all 'hard' sciences.

E: My story is that like you I was streamed into science at school, but I continued in my own right to pursue the arts and humanities. I think my mind was set to explore comfortably within both paradigms. But I do have a sense of 'belonging' within the interpretive paradigm.

N: I had been conditioned into the positivist paradigm without ever having a name for it. Is this the dominant paradigm in research today?

E: I think it is changing. The impact of critical paradigm research, feminist research and, more recently, postmodern research, suggests that pos-itivist research alone no longer holds the floor. Qualitative research is increasingly seen as acceptable to funding bodies and promotion committees.

N: The positivist paradigm seems rather too oversimplified and limited as a framework for understanding the complexity of today's world and its people.

E: Yes and no. Tradition has placed the positivist paradigm first in science and maths, yet life itself is about understanding and interpretation of phenomena, not just the collection and counting of data. And you are right; the positivist paradigm's predominately objective stance, where the data determine the answers, does appear too *neat*.

A significant challenge to the authority of the positivist paradigm comes from the works of phenomenologists such as Husserl, Heidegger, Sartre and Merleau-Ponty. For example, in *Being and Time,* Heidegger 'developed hermeneutic phenomenology as a philosophical methodology to uncover the meaning of being of human beings, the significance of which he claims had been covered over by past philosophical approaches that were reductionist and objectifying' (Plager, 1994, p. 65). The comparison between positivist and interpretive paradigm goals is summed up in the following by Wildemuth (1993, p. 451):

> It is true that the positivist approach, with its goal of discerning the statistical regularity of behavior, is oriented towards counting the occurrences and measuring the extent of the behavior being studied. By contrast, the interpretive approach, with its goal of understanding the social world from the viewpoint of the actors within it, is oriented toward detailed description of the actors' cognitive and symbolic actions, that is, the meaning associated with observable behaviors.

Lost in space

Having begun the qualitative research journey, many novice (and expert) researchers get lost. There are several good reasons for this. One is idealistic commitment to a particular research paradigm.

'Qualitative or quantitative?' – the wrong question

E: In looking at the question of whether to do qualitative versus quantitative research you are actually looking at the wrong question. It isn't whether you want to do qualitative or quantitative research (or what the terms actually mean), but where you are coming from, what paradigm you are working from, how you conceptualize knowledge and the purpose of research. It is not a question of qualitative versus quantitative.

The research question dictates what paradigm the research should be located in, not preferences to do something one way or the other. People may well be inclined to ask the sorts of question that are best answered in the qualitative paradigm, and therefore end up doing that sort of research, but the question comes first.

N: I wanted to gain an understanding of qualitative or interpretive research and so I began to read whatever I could get on the topic. I immersed myself in books for weeks and tried to gain a clear picture of what the discipline was about, but felt at the end an almost greater sense of confusion than when I began. I felt that at times the literature was actually contradictory and at times misleading.

E: Novice researchers often get lost in the literature on interpretive research. It's conceptually dense, can be conceptually foreign, and has conflicting use of terminology. As you have experienced, novice researchers often start with a limited or confused view of the paradigm, and then through the reflexive process of doing the research, gathering data, analysing, and continued reading come to a more mature and clear understanding. They also develop new understandings of the field through working towards new understandings of their data.

When considering the research, methodologies need to be selected in relation to their strengths and weaknesses and their alignment with the research question and the researcher's paradigm (or proposed paradigm); they should not be made to fit some prescribed pattern of research. Dig below the methodologies and look for the dominant and/or subservient paradigms! It therefore becomes more a question of paradigms and not methodologies. Higgs and Cant (1998, p. 1) suggest that:

> *it is important to note that neither term (qualitative and quantitative research) is fully satisfactory since in both cases qualitative and value-laden judgements can be used and interpretations are made of observations and findings.*

> *Similarly, researchers functioning within the qualitative (interpretive and critical) research paradigms can utilize quantitative techniques to analyse data. With this in mind some would argue that it is desirable to describe research approaches also in terms of the paradigm which forms the context for the research.*

Moving our focus away from the labels to some extent negates the old quantitative/qualitative argument; the labels become irrelevant as we shift our focus to the epistemological and ontological factors that underpin our paradigms.

Yet despite the realization that the qualitative/quantitative dualism is passé, it appears that the gap is widening, not closing, despite attempts to 'close it down' (Smith and Heshusius, 1986). Tellez (1998, p.1) suggests that:

> *it seems that some of those who study human behaviour have reached an uneasy truce, yet for some researchers it appears that the division is deeper than ever. Educational researchers, in particular, have now developed two separate lines of research, often existing in the same department, battling for graduate students who will use their methods.*

The question we should be asking is not whether qualitative or quantitative research is *better,* but what is our conceptual framework and within what paradigm are we working. We need to look deeper than the labels, as Olson (1996, p. 1) suggests:

> *Specific methods, particular data gathering methods, are not necessarily linked with one set of assumptions as opposed to another. The question underlying differences of research stances (or paradigms) should be their ontological and epistemological assumptions.*

Living with ambiguity/multiple paradigms

N: What happens when two conflicting paradigms compete within our thoughts? Does one paradigm overrule the other, or are we only capable of holding one paradigm at a time?

E: People who can argue or rationalize different viewpoints have an enviable gift in that they can function within multiple paradigms. They do not need to adhere to one paradigm or another; the skill lies in the ability to view life through different paradigms as required.

N: It sounds like the Orwellian notion of 'Doublethink'![1]

Many authors, including Bawden and Hames, use the analogy of 'windows in the world' to describe our personal paradigms (Bawden, 1997; Hames, 1995). Our world views are a result of many important factors – our upbringing, religious beliefs, gender, work ethics, etc. To look at the world through a different view is not to deny our values or faith, but simply to utilize our intelligence to 'put ourselves in someone else's shoes' (Hames, 1995, p. 143).

When we start looking critically at our own and conflicting paradigms, we discover we can take advantage of them all to gain different perspectives on the world. This capacity is an incredibly powerful tool in both our academic and our personal life. The ability to understand where others are coming from and how they construct their thoughts allows us to gain a better understanding of them and ourselves as well. 'Sadly, we tend to find great difficulty in stepping outside of our "tacit systems" of meaning to analyse them for what they are' (Hames, 1995, p. 147).

N: It was not until my postgraduate years that I began to understand the different types of paradigm that influence our praxis.[2] I have come to realize that it is empowering to be able to understand each paradigm; in fact, the ability to maintain multiple paradigms is a very powerful place to be!

E: As an experienced researcher, I feel quite happy to work in both paradigms, depending on my questions. But, like you, I tend more often to ask questions that lead to an interpretive paradigm.

Signposts and speed limits?

Dealing with rules and regulations – myths, legends and guidelines

N: The frames of reference and the paradigm should be considered first, but what I find is there still seems to be a number of rules and regulations I have to follow. Why? I thought that my thesis would be my story, in my words, original and innovative! Being innovative and original (at first glance) does not appear to fit in with the rigidity associated with rules and regulations.

E: Novice interpretive researchers often begin thinking they can do what they like, because a superficial reading of interpretive research makes it look so easy and creative. They fail to get to the parts of the texts that emphasize the notions of rigour, credibility and authenticity. To meet those criteria, certain rules do need to be followed, and the processes of data gathering, analysis and interpretation need to be made transparent. This trying to create order out of chaos is challenging.

McIntyre (1988, p. 161) suggests that:

> *the task of arguing methodology is one of the major accomplishments demanded by formal or academic research, and postgraduate research students who are required to defend their methodological choices often encounter difficulties in doing so. The choice of a qualitative methodology seems to exacerbate the difficulties, partly because there is a remarkable ambiguity and incoherence in the resources available for the task.*

E: In addition to the problems of ambiguity and incoherence there is also considerable breadth in interpretive research, further exacerbating the confusion that the novice experiences.

N: So the presumptions that:

- one cannot mix methodologies or use conflicting ones
- the methodology is separate from the research and researcher
- one has one's methodology clearly defined before embarking on the research
- the research fits the methodology
- research is a linear process

are more about blindly following rules, whereas we should be considering them really as guidelines; more like signposts indicating where to go than speed limits imposing rigid restrictions upon us. After all, the main rule is about knowing when to break the rules!

E: Yet the following and breaking of rules need to be true to the paradigm. My view would be that as long as you meet the quality criteria, such as rigour, authenticity and credibility, as long as you make your processes transparent, and as long as they are congruent, then you can be creative in breaking new ground and finding new ways of doing research.

N: I found that my research did not go smoothly: it was chaotic at times. How do you follow the rules and explore new grounds simultaneously? Are they not mutually exclusive?

E: Not at all! In fact, you will find this conflict more and more in interpretive research. Angela Brew (1988, p. 29) aptly describes this situation. She writes:

> *my doctoral thesis illustrates the dilemma examined in this chapter: how can we invent new methodologies for research and new forms of expression while at the same time being academically rigorous and respectable? The aim here is to address a number of issues associated with exploring ideas which are outside or on the margins of conventional definitions of acceptability in terms of methodology or knowledge. This is particularly problematic in interdisciplin-*

ary work or when we wish to explore an original methodology, engage in a meta-level critique of traditional approaches to research or question the nature of knowledge in a particular discipline.

E: In fact the relative lack of presumptions in qualitative research is both a blessing and a curse. For, paradoxically, within the confusion and lack of definite direction there is the freedom to explore emergent processes and become immersed in the rich complexity of living human phenomena.

E: I think the 'soft science' label has been given to interpretive research because readers and critics have failed to realize the rigour involved in this type of research. Of course, it's also the case that there is sloppy interpretive research around, as well as good interpretive research where the researchers have failed to report their methods in sufficient detail. The reader can be left with a sense of not trusting the data or the interpretations. Trustworthiness is an important aspect for novice interpretive researchers to understand.

Trustworthiness is a concept that embraces aspects of credibility, transferability, confirmability and dependability (Guba and Lincoln, 1994). According to Leininger, credibility refers to the truth, value or believability of findings as 'known, experienced, or deeply felt by the people being studied' (Leininger, 1994, p. 105). Confirmability refers to the obtaining of repeated evidence through participation, observation and participant feedback on findings. Transferability refers to the degree to which particular findings from an interpretive study 'can be transferred to another similar context or situation and still preserve the particularized meanings, interpretations, and inferences' (Leininger, 1994, p. 106). According to Koch, dependability can be ensured by providing a written audit trail or decision trail (Koch, 1994).

E: If interpretive researchers do all they can to establish trustworthiness, they can still exercise creativity and subjectivity. In fact, interpretive research requires creativity and flexibility during the process of data collection, in order to accommodate the unpredictability of human behaviours and capitalize on the unexpected.

Janesick (1994) has referred to this need for ongoing adjustment in her writing about 'the dance' of qualitative research design. This dance requires subtle adjustments to be made to accommodate all partners' (the researchers and their collaborators) interests and needs. In doing so, an element of subjectivity arises, but as long as it is made clear, it should be seen as a valuable part of the research process.

The researcher/research separation

N: What about the suggestion that the researcher and the research are independent? Objectivity is axiomatic in quantitative research but does not appear to be so with qualitative research. In fact there is a constant debate about the role of the researcher and the research. Do we have to remove the researcher from the research before it is regarded as valid? In 'scientific' research (within the positivist paradigm) this might have been the case, but what of qualitative research? Heshusius suggests that social scientists 'in borrowing methodology from the natural sciences in an attempt to become a "science", ... borrowed much more than methods: we borrowed the idea (not the fact, the idea) that the knower is separate from the known' (Heshusius, 1998, p. 3).

N: Are the researcher and the research interdependent in interpretive research?

E: Well, yes. The researcher is engaged in a dance with the data, moving between using his or her experience to help interpret the data (being subjective) and a desire to let the data tell its own stories (being objective). Some interpretive researchers consider researchers to be among the research tools. It is their sensitivity to the data and life experience and knowledge that enables them to respond to and interpret the data. I now understand from my experience with interpretive research what it means for the researcher to be 'a research tool'. My wealth of experience of the phenomenon under study in my PhD was both facilitative and a hindrance. It was a hindrance in that sometimes I assumed I knew what my participants were talking about and did not question further, losing opportunities for gathering valuable insights from the participants. However, my experience at other times was invaluable in alerting me to probe beneath the surface of what was being said and done, and in analysing and presenting my data. For myself as a data collecting and data analysing tool, this dance of moving between objectivity and subjectivity is deeply challenging and satisfying.

E: There is another level of interdependence to consider in interpretive research, that of the interdependent relationship between the research participants and the researcher. They jointly construct the meaning of the phenomenon under study. Discussing emergent concepts in the data and asking the participants to clarify and elaborate is one way of achieving this construction, as is asking participants to comment on the preliminary write-ups of data. In the case of my research, it involved asking my participants to comment on the narratives of experience I wrote for them. Responding to their comments in a way that preserved the 'objectivity' of my analysis and theorizing, whilst acknowledging their subjective experience of the phenomenon and now my interpretation of that, was in itself another dance.

Rothwell (1988, p. 21) suggests that the:

> *. . . traditional model regards method as the means for data collection. In fact method is the way we can guarantee the objectivity and the reliability of the data so collected. Without the application of the method no such guarantee is possible. In hermeneutical and in qualitative research there is an interplay between method and findings. In much of this research the method can be seen both as a means for guidance of data collection and as a process evolving from the data. There is a circularity here that is referred to as the* hermeneutical circle. *What is rather more important than method for the hermeneutic approach is the issue we wish to examine and analyse.*

Reason (1994, p. 16) suggests:

. . . participation is not simply a matter of interpersonal skills or political con-stitution – although these are important – it is also about the foundations of human understanding.

Experimenting

N: What if my research doesn't fit my chosen method? Is it time (to borrow from another well known science fiction series) 'to boldly go where no-one has gone before'?

E: Yes. The methodologies and methods seem to be charted territory in some ways. It's how we combine them, and how we develop and com-bine data analysis and presentation methods, that lead us into new ter-ritory. A further aspect of being a space cadet is trying out different things, different approaches to analysis and presentation, 'mining' the data in different ways, in order to capture the richness and depth of meaning. For example, I had two false starts to analysis. The first attempt at storying was rejected because it was too analytical and superficial and didn't capture the feeling of the experience, or conceptualize the experi-ence. The second attempt at analysis was grounded theory. I tried it to get at the depth of concepts and relationships in the data but I aban-doned it because I couldn't figure out how to do it on my own. The texts do not make the process transparent. I really felt I was 'lost in space' with this approach. I also felt that I was losing the affective elements and the storied aspects of the experience of my participants. Eventually, I made up my own approach, which was unique but congruent with the para-digm. The excerpts below from my thesis capture this experimentation.

I began data analysis with immersion in the data, reading and rereading the transcripts of the interviews collected from the first two participants. The aim was to create a general framework for codes to be applied to chunking and coding of the transcript data as described by Miles and Huberman (1993). Although such a framework was developed, it failed to capture the reflective and dynamic nature of lived experience. Titchen and McIntyre identified a similar difficulty in using this approach to data analysis, reporting that the 'excessive detail and incoherence of the cod-ing frame' (Titchen and McIntyre, 1993, p. 33) did not convey the ways in which their participants were making sense out of their experiences nor the logic which lay behind their words and actions.

Further, the coding framework which I developed failed to capture the affective domain of experience and the growth and development experi-enced by the clinical educators and described of the students. The tem-poral dimension of lived experience was also elusive. Goodfellow (1995) experienced similar difficulties in her preliminary coding of data collected through observation and interview of preschool teachers who were supervising students. She reported the criticisms by one of her partici-pants that while her analysis 'represented "the ideal" it did not represent "reality" to him' (p. 75). Goodfellow found herself 'trying to deal with the data in a way which was in conflict with the temporality and sequen-tiality of experience itself' (p. 75). A different approach to data analysis was called for; one which would capture the reflective, logical and dynamic nature of the lived experience of the clinical educators in the study.

It's important to note that in this experimentation I followed the guidelines for establishing trustworthiness and credibility. I believe you have to be able to justify what you do, not just go down any path that attracts you. It's that notion of applying 'rigour' in interpretive research.

Splashdown!

N: I found after re-reading our correspondence and reflections that I did not feel totally 'lost in space' and that there was some order in the chaos. This feeling of relief had the effect of liberating me from my self-doubt and gave me a feeling of 'WOW' that was quite exhilarating! The rules, regulations and guidelines that I thought were prescriptive and binding were paradoxically part of the very framework that supports my journey.

E: There have been several times during the process of my first major interpretive study where I have felt totally lost, drowning in data, confused by the lack of explanation and guidance on how to actually undertake interpretive analyses, paralysed into inactivity by anxiety about whether what I was doing was 'right' or made sense or was rigorous enough or intellectually defensible. The self-doubt and plummeting self-esteem has been cyclical, as I enter each new phase of the study and write up. The consequent procrastination has been annoying but wryly amusing. I laughed with glee and a sense of self-affirmation when I read the Ely *et al.* (1991) book, where Ely courageously recounts scrubbing her bathroom tiling with a toothbrush (to remove mould) rather than face her current qualitative research project. I had only a couple of days earlier done just the same thing, and was wondering whether this 'damned qualitative research' was driving me crazy!

Moustakis has outlined five phases in qualitative research, which are quite helpful in understanding the cycles of qualitative research and the emotional merry-go-round that accompanies the process. The phases are immersion in the setting (and data), incubation, illumination, explication, and creative synthesis (Moustakis, 1990). Morse discusses how 'as the study progresses, theoretical insights and linkages between categories increase, making the process exciting as "what is going on" finally becomes clearer and more obvious' (Morse, 1994, p. 230).

E: I think the phases outlined by Moustakis are cyclical and that we may revisit some or all of them as we commence each new stage of our interpretive study. I would suggest that excitement and anticipation accompany the initial phase of immersion, soon to be followed by a sense of being overwhelmed by the amount of data and ambiguities in the setting. Looking at the next stage as 'incubation' is a positive reframing for the sense of 'not being able to move forward' that sometimes follows. Much thinking and ruminating occurs in this phase, often with little tangible evidence until you begin to write. The final phase of creative synthesis is often revealed in the outpouring of writing that follows periods of feeling 'lost in space'. That phase is truly exhilarating, when you find yourself writing with insight, illuminating your data and explicating your emergent theory, and making links perhaps not consciously considered prior to the act of writing. You finally come to what Morse described as knowing what is going on. The creative synthesis that emerges makes the periods of incubation and self-questioning seem worthwhile. There is a sense of WOW – did I really think this/write this?

That sense of WOW also came for me from realizing that whilst I had followed the rules about ensuring rigour, I had indeed come up with a unique methodology, which combined existing methodologies and applied them to a new context. It's affirming to realize that my cycles of self-doubt, feeling like a space cadet and lost in space, have finally resulted in new and worthwhile insights into my profession. When presented at conferences, the stories of the experience of being a clinical educator resonate with clinical educators in the audience, who say they feel understood and valued. The theoretical modelling I believe has value in preparing and supporting clinical educators in their role.

N: I like your interpretation of Moustakis' phases as being cyclic in nature and the fact that we may revisit them at certain stages of our journey. I would also add another cyclic analogy in the interpretation of my studies. At times I feel like a spinning top, the type we probably played with as kids; as I cycle through from lost in space to insight, then on to 'WOW', I sometimes lose momentum and my spin begins to wobble. It takes only a small 'push' or 'wow' to give me impetus again. This impetus might come from a sudden insight, an affirmation, a dialogue such as this or personal reflections and self-motivation.

This dialogue has reminded me that my journey is one that is not perfectly mapped out, and that at times I will have to backtrack to re-find my way. It has reinforced the fact that there are rules to be followed (and occasionally bent) and the fact that there are 'wows' to be had, along with the frustration, hard work and adventure that a learning journey such as this entails.

Summary

In this chapter we have used the device of dialogue between a novice and a more experienced (slightly less novice, anyway!) interpretive researcher to highlight some of the trials and tribulations inherent in being a methodological space cadet within this paradigm. Through our dialogue and our reflections on the literature, we have considered the pitfalls in learning to do interpretive research. It is rarely the clear-cut, linear process the literature would have us believe. In part this is due to the nature of the research: each interpretive project is unique, and to attempt to apply a set of rules to the endeavour is antithetical to the nature of interpretive inquiry. In addition, however, the anguish of the interpretive paradigm space cadet is due in part to the lack of detail and transparency of the processes reported in published research. Having taken the bold step of engaging in such research ought perhaps lead to courage in revealing the pitfalls and flaws of the research process in the write-up phase. Now that interpretive research has, through the efforts of methodological pioneers, gained respectability in most academic circles, let us hope that the increasing number of books and research reports in the area might make more transparent the processes for the new generation of space cadets.

[1] 'Doublethink means the power of holding two contradictory beliefs in one's mind simultaneously, and accepting both of them' (Orwell, 1949, p. 9).

[2] In this work we have taken praxis to mean 'the application of a theory to cases encountered in experience, but is also ethically significant thought, or practical reason' (Blackburn, 1994, p. 298).

References

Bawden, R. (1997) The community challenge: the learning response. Invited plenary paper to 29th Annual International Meeting of the Community Development Society. Athens, GA, 27–30 July.

Blackburn, S. (1994) *The Oxford Dictionary of Philosophy*. Oxford: Oxford University Press.

Brew, A. (1988) Moving beyond paradigm boundaries. In *Writing Qualitative Research* (J. Higgs, ed.), pp. 29–46. Sydney: Hampden Press.

Denzin, N. and Lincoln, Y. (eds) (1994) *Handbook of Qualitative Research*. Thousand Oaks: Sage.

Ely, M., Anzul, M., Friedman, T., Garner, D. and Steinmetz, A. (1991) *Doing Qualitative Research: Circles Within Circles*. London: The Falmer Press.

Goodfellow, J. (1995) Cooperating teachers' images: a study in early childhood settings. Unpublished PhD thesis, The University of Sydney, NSW, Australia.

Guba, E. G. and Lincoln, Y. S. (eds) (1994) *Competing Paradigms in Qualitative Research*. Thousand Oaks: Sage.

Hames, R. D. (1995) *The Management Myth*. Sydney: Business and Professional Publishing.

Heshusius, L. (1998) *Methodological Concerns Around Subjectivity: Will We Free Ourselves From Objectivity?* http://www.irn.pdx.edu/~kerlinb/qualresearch/Heshusius.html (27/12/98).

Higgs, J. (1998) Structuring qualitative research theses. In *Writing Qualitative Research* (J. Higgs, ed.), pp. 151–160. Sydney: Hampden Press.

Higgs, J. and Cant, R. (1998) What is qualitative research? In *Writing Qualitative Research* (J. Higgs, ed.), pp. 1–8. Sydney: Hampden Press.

Janesick, V. (1994) The dance of qualitative research design: metaphor, methodolatory, and meaning. In *Handbook of Qualitative Research* (N. Denzin and Y. Lincoln, eds), pp. 209–219. Thousand Oaks: Sage.

Koch, T. (1994) Establishing rigor in qualitative research: The decision trail. *Journal of Advanced Nursing*, **19**, 976–986.

Leininger, M. (1994) Evaluation criteria and critique of qualitative studies. In *Critical Issues in Qualitative Research Methods* (J. M. Morse, ed.), pp. 95–115. Thousand Oaks: Sage.

McAllister, L. (2001) What's it like to be a clinical educator?: a phenomenological study of the experience of being a clinical educator. Unpublished PhD thesis, The University of Sydney, NSW, Australia.

McIntyre, J. (1988) Arguing for an interpretive method. In *Writing Qualitative Research* (J. Higgs, ed.), pp. 161–174. Sydney: Hampden Press.

Miles, M. and Huberman, A. (1993) *Qualitative Data Analysis: A Sourcebook of New Methods*. Newbury Park: Sage.

Mills, I. (1994) *When Our Lips Speak Together–Part one*. The Faculty of Health, Humanities and Social Ecology, University of Western Sydney, NSW, Australia.

Morse, J. (1994) Designing funded qualitative research. In *Handbook of Qualitative Research* (N. Denzin and Y. Lincoln, eds), pp. 220–235. Thousand Oaks: Sage.

Moustakis, C. (1990) *Heuristic Research Design, Methodology, and Applications.* Newbury Park: Sage.

Olson, H. (1996) *Quantitative 'Versus' Qualitative Research: The Wrong Question.* http://www.ualberta.ca/dept/slis/cais/olson.html (08/10/96).

Orwell, G. (1949) *Animal Farm.* London: Penguin Books.

Pippen, E. (1998) *Stand by to Raise Ship!!* http://www.solarguard.com/sghome.htm (11/11/98).

Plager, K. (1994) Hermeneutic phenomenology. In *Interpretive Phenomenology* (P. Benner, ed.), pp. 65–84. Thousand Oaks: Sage.

Reason, P. (ed.) (1994) *Participation in Human Inquiry.* London: Sage.

Rothwell, R. (1988) Philosophical paradigms and qualitative research. In *Writing Qualitative Research* (J. Higgs, ed.), pp. 21–28. Sydney: Hampden Press.

Smith, J. K. and Heshusius, L. (1986) Closing down the conversation: the end of the quantitative–qualitative debate among educational researchers. *Educational Researcher*, **15**(1), 4–12.

Tellez, K. (1998) *The Legend of the Qualitative/Quantitative Dualism: Implications for Research in Technology and Teacher Education.* http://www.coe.uh.edu/~ktellez/qqte.html (27/12/98).

Titchen, A. and McIntyre, D. (1993) A phenomenological approach to qualitative data analysis in nursing research. In *Changing Nursing Practice Through Action Research* (A. Titchen, ed.), pp. 29–48. Oxford: National Institute for Nursing Centre for Practice Development.

Wildemuth, B. M. (1993) Post-positivist research: two examples of methodological pluralism. *Library Quarterly*, **63**, 450–468.

4

Charting standpoints in qualitative research

Joy Higgs

Are we as qualitative researchers lost in the space and time of postmodernity? In this chapter I propose a (meta-) framework (or a dynamic coherent frame of reference being continually reconstructed by the researcher). I use the analogy of time and space travellers charting their direction through uncertain territory and dimensions by using the stars and other points of reference, and adopting standpoints of operational and philosophical principles (also called philosophical stances) as 'prime directives' to guide and frame the journey. Crotty (1998a, p. 183) took a similar approach when he pondered the question: 'Postmodernism: Crisis of confidence or moment of truth?'. He generated a scaffold to support and structure research for the seeker of direction amidst the confusion of postmodern research.

My framework comprises five metaphors to reflect critical moments in the research journey. At these points immersion in being lost, confused or overwhelmed is just as important a part of learning the craft and inspiration of research as are the moments of clarity when decisions, realizations and elevations to a higher plane of understanding seem to fall readily into place. *Being lost in space and time* considers the challenges that qualitative researchers can encounter in the face of a burgeoning but confusing array of research methodologies and criteria for quality evaluation within a postmodern era. *Framing the research journey* examines ways different frameworks and frames of reference can facilitate the research process. *Dancing on the carpet* is a metaphor which recognizes the value of knowing and enjoying existing theoretical foundations that support new research adventures. *Illuminating the phenomenon* illustrates the goal, the challenge and the wonder of discovering and of extending knowledge in our chosen topic area. Finally, *conversing with peers and sages* recognizes the task of the researcher to present the research proposal and (emerging) findings for scrutiny, to argue the case convincingly and not to be intimidated by articulate members of the dominant research paradigm.

Being lost in space and time

Qualitative researchers today face several challenges. What is the difference between qualitative and quantitative research? Is survey research qualitative? (It appears to be so in the minds of people sending theses out for examination, regardless of whether the results are quantified, statistically analysed and presented numerically in detailed tables seeking to present a population sample. Perhaps education is the key factor missing in this conclusion.) Is qualitative research the poor cousin: never considered good enough, never likely to win the prizes (grants, scholarships, etc.), never likely to progress the researcher's career as well as the dominant quantitative research approach does. These questions are located among terminological, educational, political and preference issues. The following quotation from Edwards' (1997) thesis illustrates a number of the issues that qualitative researchers have faced, and continue to encounter in many arenas:

> *As this study is being written up in the 1990s, adopting a qualitative paradigm in educational research is not unusual. Nor is it considered necessary to defend it at length against the positivistic arguments of the quantitative paradigm. However, when the fieldwork began in the early 1980s quite a different situation prevailed. The qualitative tradition was just beginning to appear in mainstream educational research, especially in the area of evaluation. Pioneers, such as Parlett and Hamilton (1972) who wrote of 'illuminative' evaluation and Guba (1978) of 'naturalistic' evaluation, began publishing in limited-circulation monographs. During the later 1980s there was a huge growth in approaches to educational research and evaluation based on the qualitative paradigm, to the extent that Fetterman (1988) used the phrase 'a silent scientific revolution in evaluation' in a book title to describe the extent of the expansion of qualitative methods.*

> *Yet, the revolution was not always silent. For much of the 1980s the qualitative approach was attacked by quantitative researchers, mainly on the grounds of what they saw as lack of methodological rigour. A polarized debate developed, particularly in the United States, which emphasized differences rather than complementarity. Quantitative research was portrayed as factual and value-free while qualitative research was seen as value-laden. Some writers, for example Howe (1985, 1988), attempted to defuse the debate by suggesting that the factual versus value-judgement, and positivistic versus interpretivistic debate was no longer an issue in the post-positive conception of the world portrayed by writers such as Quine, Kuhn and Scriven (Howe, 1985): indeed this researcher would agree with such a position. Other writers, for example Smith and Heshusius (1986), were not so comfortable with the emerging accommodation between the two paradigms. They argued that 'the claim of compatibility, let alone one of synthesis, cannot be sustained' (Smith and Heshusius, 1986, p. 4). They suggest that 'closing down the conversation' of the quantitative/qualitative debate detracts from our basic understanding of what we do as inquirers.*

Understanding qualitative research – understanding and choosing your standpoint

No researcher can ignore the politics of advancement and hegemony. However, there are more critical questions needing to be asked to help us focus on how, what, where and with whom to research, including the following: Where am I coming from? What is my philosophical stance? What do I want to research? What is my personal frame of reference? What am I seeking to achieve? (In what way) am I trying to make a difference? What standards should I be addressing to ensure that in choosing qualitative research I am indeed making a quality contribution to knowledge?

Let us consider first the notion of what qualitative research is. Even though we have chosen the term for the title of this book, the word itself is problematic. It has been used more as a rallying point for people who are willing to look beyond the dominant quantitative/experimental research paradigm or who find the restrictions of this powerful research system too great. One of the issues we are addressing in this book is the need for 'and': for qualitative as well as quantitative research, given the range of questions that many fields of research encounter. To address this issue let me first provide a simple definition of qualitative research; that is, *research which relies on qualitative (non-mathematical) judgments*. However, this distinction is not a straightforward matter. Consider the depth of issues inherent in the assumptions underpinning different research approaches.

Lincoln and Guba (1985), for instance, provide an analysis of the five major assumptions about the construction and nature of knowledge that underpin qualitative and quantitative research. These assumptions characterize qualitative research as a constructivist approach in which findings, shaped by multiple realities, emerge as the research proceeds, through interaction between the investigator and subjects or respondents.

- Qualitative research assumes that the world consists of 'multiple constructed realities'. 'Multiple' implies that there are always several versions of reality, depending on from which or whose perspective it is viewed. 'Constructed' means that participants attribute meaning to events as they occur; that meaning is part of the event and not separate from it.
- Qualitative research assumes that the process of inquiry changes both the investigator and the subject: that the investigator and the subject are interdependent. This assumption is in contrast to the 'independence' of research and researcher demanded by quantitative research.
- A third assumption relates to the nature of knowledge. Whereas quantitative research seeks generalizations and universal truths, qualitative research maintains that knowledge is both time and context dependent. Rather than searching for generalizations, qualitative research looks for 'a deep understanding of the particular' (Domholdt, 1993, p. 127).
- Qualitative research holds that it is useful to describe and interpret events in order to answer some research questions, rather than to control events in an attempt to establish cause and effect.
- Qualitative inquiry is 'value bound': it is seen as impossible to separate value from inquiry; values are revealed in the way questions are asked and results interpreted.

Choosing a method – making a meaningful choice or taking a lucky dip?

Apart from trying to understand what qualitative research is all about, novice researchers and, indeed, experienced researchers new to qualitative research are both faced with two other areas of confusion: the huge array of methodologies which appear to fall under this title, and the considerable confusion linked to what constitutes good qualitative research.

A variety of approaches have been produced to conceptualize or categorize approaches within the qualitative paradigm. Tesch (1992) described rapid growth in qualitative approaches, tracing their roots to psychology, sociology, education and anthropology. She described the resulting proliferation of qualitative approaches as confusion and overlap of philosophies, methods and terms. Tesch distinguishes among a number of different qualitative approaches, and relates these approaches to research questions. Other categorizations have been developed by Bogdan and Bilken (1992) and Denzin and Lincoln (1994). One of the challenges facing qualitative researchers is to find convincing quality assurance strategies. Such strategies need to maintain the freedom qualitative research has gained from the reductionism and restrictions in choice of question in quantitative research and avoid the traps that could arise in the face of the new rules and prescriptiveness that are creeping into qualitative research.

There is a growing tendency in some areas to insist upon precise criteria being addressed for research to be recognized as belonging to specific types of qualitative research and to be considered sound research. Instead of falling into this new prescriptive trap, let me propose the following guidelines for achieving quality in process and product of qualitative research:

- understand the origins and canons of your selected research approach and endeavour to adopt research design, implementation, evaluation and reporting strategies which are true to/congruent with that approach
- where your chosen strategy involves the blending of two approaches, use your depth of understanding of these approaches to plan and implement research activities which address these combined goals and expectations (e.g. understanding and enabling change)
- read widely and adopt an approach which is compatible with your personal frame of reference (including your values, aspirations, self-image, etc.), and acknowledge the derivation of your approach. When the original researcher's approach is not adopted specifically it is preferable to describe your design using phrases like 'informed by van Manen's approach to hermeneutic phenomenology' rather than 'using van Manen's hermeneutic phenomenology approach'
- identify the criteria for assessing your research which you (a) consider to be credible as benchmarks of quality for your selected approach, (b) will apply consistently during the research, and (c) will use to assess the achieved quality of your work
- realize the limits of one person's experience and seek comment on your work (design, process and product) from experienced people (with content and/or method expertise). Research students are unwise to rely only on their supervisor(s). Other research advisors can enrich the research and provide valuable troubleshooting or alternate perspectives.

Framing the research journey – developing research maps

Framing our research journeys involves several factors, including matching goals and strategies, understanding paradigms, addressing the issue of credibility by embedding the research in methodological understanding, and creating a coherent research framework.

Matching goals and strategies

The following thesis extract (Edwards, 1997) illustrates the task of the researcher to match research goals and strategies:

> *In recent years there has been a growing perception that researchers, who are supposed to feed the professional schools with useful knowledge, have less and less to say that practitioners find useful (Schön, 1987, p. 10). It was the intention in this study to go a small way to meeting such criticisms by contributing to, and developing, knowledge which could be useful for clinical teachers in health professions. The project investigated, analysed and described a largely unresearched aspect of clinical teaching and learning; specifically, the content and process of, and influences on, the day-to-day interactions between teachers and students in clinical settings. In order to achieve this, a qualitative research paradigm was adopted, a naturalistic interpretative approach was taken to data collection, and an inductive interpretative process adopted for data analysis and presentation of results.*

Understanding research paradigms and philosophical underpinnings

Research paradigms can be used to reduce some of the confusion that exists when we use the terms qualitative and quantitative research. In this chapter these terms are replaced by three research paradigm labels: the empirico-analytical, interpretive and critical research paradigms. Philosophical frameworks or research paradigms contain different ontological (worldview) and epistemological (knowledge derivation) perspectives on knowledge (see Table 4.1). To this is added a fourth way of knowing: the creative arts paradigm. (For further discussion on this topic see Higgs *et al.*, 2001a, and Titchen and Higgs, 2001.)

Research seeks to generate knowledge. Understanding forms of knowledge and the manner of generation and verification of knowledge is an important part of the research process and of the researcher's role in transforming research questions into defensible knowledge claims.

Vico (1668–1744) categorized knowledge as deductive (knowledge by definition), scientific (knowledge from empirical evidence) and experiential (knowledge from personal experience) (Berlin, 1979).

- *Deductive knowledge* takes certain propositions or assumptions as a starting point and follows where those assumptions logically lead. Vico referred to this knowledge as things that are true either by definition or by deduction from other things that are themselves true purely by definition.
- *Scientific knowledge* requires objectively valid, reliable and reproducible evidence. And only evidence gained by the senses – through observation, description and measurement – may be counted. Knowledge remains 'true' only for as long as it is not objectively refuted; when it fails that crucial test it becomes obsolete, to be replaced by a superior formula.
- *Experiential knowledge* is gained by personal experience. Some crucially important human knowledge exists, Vico argued, which is distinct from and not reducible to either scientific or deductive knowledge.

A related approach developed to characterize professional knowledge (Higgs and Titchen, 1995) includes propositional knowledges (derived

Table 4.1 Research paradigms (based on Higgs and Titchen, 1995, 2001). See Table 4.2 for definition of key terms

Ontology

deals with what exists, what is reality, what is the nature of the world. It is concerned with the study of existence itself and differentiates between 'real existence' and 'appearance' (Flew, 1984). Researchers need to understand the assumptions about existence underlying any theory or system of ideas we use to research and interpret the world.

Epistemology

deals with how what exists may be known. 'Central issues in epistemology are the nature and derivation of knowledge, the scope of knowledge, and the reliability of claims to knowledge' (Flew, 1984, p. 109).

The empirico-analytical paradigm

is based on positivist or empiricist philosophy and employs the scientific method of inquiry. This approach is adopted in the natural sciences and relies on observation and experiment in the empirical world, resulting in generalizations about the content and events of the world which can be used to predict future experience (Moore, 1982). In the *empirico-analytical paradigm*, knowledge:

- is discovered, i.e. universal and external truths are grasped and justified
- arises from empirical processes which are reductionist, value neutral, quantifiable, objective and operationalizable
- statements are valid only if publicly verifiable by sense data.

The interpretive paradigm

is commonly based on the philosophy of idealism. This paradigm encompasses a number of research approaches (including hermeneutics, constructivism, phenomenology and ethnography) that have the central goal of seeking to interpret the world, particularly the social world. These interpretive methodologies (e.g. Rabinow and Sullivan, 1979; MacLeod, 1990; Brown and McIntyre, 1993) offer valuable ways of studying everyday experience and practice in ways which retain experiential and contextual integrity (Higgs and Titchen, 1995). In the *interpretive paradigm*, knowledge:

- comprises constructions arising from the minds and bodies of knowing, conscious and feeling beings
- is generated through a search for meaning, beliefs and values, and through looking for wholes and relationships with other wholes.

The critical paradigm

is based on the philosophy of realism. In this epistemology, knowledge is not grasped or discovered but is acquired through critical debate (Barnett, 1990). In the *critical paradigm*, knowledge:

- is emancipatory and personally developmental
- requires becoming aware of how our thinking is socially and historically constructed and how this limits our actions
- enables people to challenge learned restrictions, compulsions or dictates of habit
- is not grasped or discovered but is acquired through critical debate
- promotes understanding about how to transform current structures, relationships and conditions which constrain development and reform.

Continued

Table 4.1 – *continued*

The creative arts paradigm
is based on embodied, spiritual, intuitive and cognitive ways of knowing which occur in the practice of the creative arts. Such ways of knowing are pertinent to professional areas beyond the creative arts including education (see Fish, 1998) and the health sciences (see Benner, 1984; Titchen, 2000). The epitome of knowing in the creative arts is professional artistry. Eisner (1985) conceived of such knowing as connoisseurship. He described it as a way of paying attention, and adopted the accompanying notion of criticism as a way of disclosing or expressing what had been seen. Similarly Fish (1998) contended that the development of professional artistry requires attention to the dimensions of practice which are often invisible, the values, beliefs, attitudes, assumptions, expectations, feelings and knowledge that lie below the surface and behind the actions of the practitioner. Professional artistry is owned by an individual who possesses a blend of qualities built up through extensive and reflective individual knowledge and experience (Beeston and Higgs, 2001). Professional expertise resides in practice wisdom and professional artistry (Higgs *et al.*, 2001b); it is a deep knowing in practice (Eraut, 1985). This argument is supported by Benner *et al.* (1996), who recognize the place of Aristotelian practical reasoning in expert clinical judgment.

from research and theory) and two forms of non-propositional knowledge, namely professional craft knowledge (arising from professional experience) and personal knowledge (arising from personal experience). This approach emphasizes how professionals derive non-propositional knowledge from both personal life experience and work experience, and how they draw on both of these forms of knowledge (as well as on propositional knowledge) in their professional work.

The importance of understanding the epistemological and ontological perspectives we adopt in research is evident in the following quotations:

Any research, whether in the natural or social sciences, makes knowledge claims and for that reason alone is implicated in epistemological questions. It could be argued that all research is based on an epistemology even though this is not always made explicit – in fact most of the time the epistemology that underlies a particular piece of research is taken for granted. It is simply assumed that the research will be positivist/empiricist in its epistemology and therefore unproblematic as an epistemology. (Usher, 1996, p. 11)

I think researchers need to know when they're setting out on research what kind of knowledge and theory they're hoping to generate as the product of the research ... unless one understands epistemology one is not clear about what different kinds of knowledge there are and what different kinds of knowledge are generated in different kinds of (research) approaches and in different paradigms. So I think understanding the research paradigm underpinning the research is absolutely essential and I think a lot of the problem with a lot of flawed research is that there isn't an understanding of epistemology and ontology. (QRP – RP1)[1]

Understanding the epistemological underpinning of a research strategy arises from contemplation of the following questions: What do I understand about how knowledge is created? In the context of the research issue, question and setting I am addressing, what view of knowledge generation is most pertinent? It could be argued, for instance, that the researcher seeking to measure the performance of a muscle under mechanical stress would set out to collect sense data to test a hypothesis, adopting the scientific method of the empirico-analytical paradigm. The human services worker seeking to understand consumers' experiences of a particular mode of service would commonly adopt an interpretive approach. By comparison, the critical paradigm would be preferred if the researcher wanted to work with a community to identify goals and strategies for changing the governing structure and regulation of that community. Table 4.2 provides an overview of a number of the most recognized ontological and epistemological perspectives.

Addressing credibility – embedding our research in methodological understanding

Next we should consider the status and credibility of qualitative research. Thorne (1997, p. 117) argues: 'despite the enthusiastic claims of its adherents that qualitative research is the key to accessing subjective realities, the products of qualitative inquiries are not inevitably accurate, relevant, or even socially responsible'. She contends that flaws in qualitative research 'are a product of an incomplete shift from a quantitative to qualitative philosophical orientation'.

The first step in countering the problem Thorne identifies is to develop a deep understanding of the alternative paradigms that have emerged alongside the quantitative (or empirico-analytical) paradigm. Table 4.3 provides an analysis of the three research paradigms identified in this chapter to represent a useful classification of research approaches. It is notable that:

- the various dimensions (see the different columns) within each research paradigm need to be congruent; they need to be coherent and make sense as a whole, to give meaning and context to the paradigm
- each paradigm has a unique philosophical underpinning which defines the stance taken by researchers in that paradigm
- it is feasible to adopt a combined approach, incorporating elements of different paradigms within a coherent philosophical and theoretical stance (e.g. working within the critical paradigm, but drawing on the interpretive paradigm, or using an interpretive feminist approach)
- methods of data collection and analysis can be adopted in more than one paradigm or approach, if they are consistent with the relevant research goals and philosophical stance
- the definitions of specifying characteristics, dimensions and evaluation criteria for the interpretive and critical paradigms have undergone a substantial shift from the quantitative philosophical and methodological orientation.

For instance, compared to the positivist philosophy of the empirico-analytical paradigm, the idealist philosophy (which provides the foundation for interpretive paradigm research) 'questions the possibility of a mind-independent world, insisting that the external material world is known through the perceptions and subjectivity of humans' (Powers and Knapp,

Table 4.2 Ontological and epistemological perspectives (Higgs and Titchen, 1998). Note: this is a simplified analysis of a complex array of perspectives. It provides a useful starting point to facilitate the exploration of other galaxies

ONTOLOGICAL PERSPECTIVES:

a) In the traditional experimental methodology '**materialist**' view, 'science is only about that which exists materially, it is not interested in the study of phenomena that are non-material ... in fact many scientists and materialist philosophers go so far as to deny the reality of non-material phenomena' (Rothwell, 1995, p. 2).

b) In the **positivist/empiricist** research tradition the world is objective, since it is said to exist independently of the knowers, and it consists of phenomena or events that are orderly and lawful.

c) In the **constructivist** view, knowers are seen as conscious subjects separate from a world of objects; subjects who use knowledge who have theories about their practice and who behave according to tacit rules and procedures. In qualitative research, in general, multiple constructed realities are recognized to occur (i.e. different people have different perceptions of reality through their attribution of meaning to events, meaning being part of the event not separate from it) (Lincoln and Guba, 1985).

d) A **social constructivist** view contends that reality and knowledge are socially constructed. That is, reality exists because we give meaning to it (Berger and Luckmann, 1985). Different cultures have different social constructions of reality. Within the **interpretive** tradition, the world and reality are interpreted by people in the context of historical and social practices.

e) A **hermeneutic** view arises from the ideas of Merleau-Ponty (1956), Heidegger (1962) and Gadamer (1975), amongst others. In this approach, knowing is seen as a kind of being, as a concrete form of being-in-the-world and as pragmatic, involved activity or 'know-how' that is more basic than, and occurs prior to, reflective thinking. This knowing is embedded in unarticulated common meanings and shared background practices of groups of people. Unlike the constructivist view of knowledge, this knowing has no mental representation and may be embodied, that is, known by the body without cognition. In this hermeneutic view, there is no subject/object split; people are seen, first and foremost, as part of the world, in amongst it, being in it, and coping with it. They are also seen as beings for whom things have significance and value, as having a world of background practices, social practices and historical contexts and as being a person in time (Leonard, 1989). This view of people and the world is a relational one (Benner and Wrubel, 1989), in which our relation to objects is not something represented in our minds.

f) In **critical theory** there is a focus on the social world: people are socially located and therefore knowledge is always influenced by social interest (see Habermas, 1972).

Table 4.2 – *continued*

EPISTEMOLOGICAL PERSPECTIVES:

a) To **positivists** or **empiricists**, knowledge arises from the rigorous application of the scientific method and is measured against the criteria of objectivity, reliability and validity.

b) The **idealist** approaches of Dilthey (1833–1911) and Weber (1864–1920) focused on interpretive understanding (*verstehen*), to accessing the ideas and experiences of actors/participants, as opposed to the explanatory and predictive approach of the physical sciences (Smith, 1983). Dilthey presented understanding as a hermeneutic process involving constant movement between parts and whole. This perspective results in a focus on human behaviour as occurring within a context, and the understanding or knowledge of human behaviour as requiring an understanding of this context.

c) **Constructivists** view knowledge as 'an internal construction or an attempt to impose meaning and significance on events and ideas. In this perspective each person constructs a more-or-less idiosyncratic explanatory system of reality' (Candy, 1991, p. 251).

d) The **social constructionist** approach (McCarthy, 1996) construes knowledge as a changing and relative phenomenon and examines the social and historical constructs of knowledge in terms of what knowledge is socially produced and what counts as knowledge.

e) The **realist** is concerned with social structures, and how macro- and micro-political, historical, and socio-economic factors influence our lives and how we understand our lives.

1995, p. 133), while in the realist philosophy (of the critical paradigm) knowledge emerges from debate and social practice. Similarly, typical qualitative research strategies (such as the following) prompt re-thinking of traditional standards.

Qualitative research demonstrates a number of commonalities (Powers and Knapp, 1995), such as:

- personal involvement between researcher and informants in the latter's natural setting
- intensive interviews with detailed description of conversations and observations
- introspection and self-reflection to provide the researcher's individual responses to the data (reflexivity)
- openness to discovery and unexpected findings
- willingness to re-direct the research on the basis of new understandings/ insights emerging from concurrent data collection and analysis
- operational and theoretical management of large volumes of descriptive data via various means.

These philosophies and strategies run counter to the constraints, expectations and gold standards of quantitative research: validity, reliability and

Table 4.3 A framework for research implementation and reporting – dimensions[+]

Internal context	External context	Philosophical stance	Research paradigm	Research goals	Research approach(es)	Research methods – data collection	Research methods – data analysis	Report writing	Quality control/review
Includes:		*Positivism* (Objectivity is the key issue, sense data determines reality)	*Empirico-analytical paradigm*	To measure, test hypotheses, discover, predict, explain, control, generalize, identify cause-effect relationships	Experimental method (The scientific method) Descriptive, comparative studies (testing hypotheses)	Controlled trials Interviews Questionnaires	Statistical analysis	Objective, structured, scholarly Decontextualized	*Objectivity, Validity, Reliability*
Individual and collective:	Research question							For headings, see French (1993), Burnard (1992)	*Rigour*
a) Personal frame(s) of reference	Theoretical framework of the topic area	*Idealism* (Emphasis is on the actors' ideas or embodied knowing as the determinant of social reality. There are multiple constructed or storied realities)	*Interpretive paradigm*	To understand, interpret, seek meaning, describe, illuminate, theorize	Hermeneutics, phenomenology, narrative inquiry, naturalistic inquiry, historiography	Interviews Case studies Story telling Review of texts, creative arts media	Repeated return to data (the process is circular, iterative, spiral) extraction of themes theorization, interpretation of texts and artworks	Contextual relational, qualitative, scholarly, rich description, can include stories, artworks, theorization	*Credibility* (incl. trustworthiness) *Soundness* (incl. authenticity and congruence) *Ethicality* *Quality writing, Valuable contribution* *Quality*
b) Knowledge base(s) of researcher(s)	Domain of research e.g. physical sciences, social sciences or both	*Realism* (Social practice and culture shape practice)	*Critical paradigm*	To improve, reform, empower, change reality or situation	Action research/collaborative research Praxis – acting on existing conditions to change them	Interviews Case studies Story telling Review of texts Critical debate Review of espoused theory vs theory in action Creative arts media	Scholarly analysis of action/effects Critical debate Review of espoused theory vs theory in action Sharing knowledge and experience Reflecting upon data collected, action and outcomes, scholarly analysis Refining/elaborating knowledge	Contextual, experiential, descriptive, reflective, critique Principles for transformative action. Can include theorization and stories, artworks Rich description	As above + The change action/strategy is deemed to be successful by the actors Existing knowledge is refined or elaborated
		Combined stances	Combined paradigms						

+ Based on Higgs (1998). Input from A. Titchen is acknowledged.

objectivity. We need to replace these measures with more relevant criteria of quality, such as credibility (see Table 4.3).

The second step in countering potential accusations of unsatisfactory qualitative research products lies in understanding the chosen approach well and implementing it credibly and authentically. This understanding can be achieved through exploration of the following questions:

- What research options are available to address my research topic/question?

For each option consider:

- What is the general tradition and paradigmatic origin of this approach?
- What are the dimensions of this approach? How is knowledge viewed? What methodologies are used?
- What forms of research does this tradition adopt? (examine some exemplars).
- What are the relative strengths and limitations of this option compared to the others being considered?
- What theoretical perspective do I want to use to frame and inform this research? Does this influence the preferred research strategy?
- Do I need to use a combination of research approaches, usually considered to be located in different paradigms? If so, how can I ensure that a congruent philosophical standpoint is adopted? (see the Titchen, 2000, extract below).

Creating a coherent research framework/research map

A coherent framework for qualitative research is an important step in providing a sense of direction as well as a fluid base for responsiveness to emerging research experiences and outcomes. Research frameworks in qualitative research need to be seen as dynamic, coherent frames of reference rather than as procedural regulations. This is illustrated by the following quote from an experienced researcher.

> *I personally find it very important to have a working framework that guides the process of the research, the data collection and the analysis ... but I don't have a strong sense that once that framework is put down on paper or in my head that it's fixed, because I feel that when you get involved in research, new questions and new thoughts come into it all the time, that it's limited not to be flexible enough to explore new avenues that come up in terms of the congruence of it all, I think it's important that there's a degree of congruence and that you're not trying to join completely opposing philosophies or starting points. But there needs to be room to explore within the framework. (QRP – RP4)*

Figure 4.1 provides a framework to guide the qualitative researcher. In fact this is a meta-framework, which includes the philosophical framework (or stance) and the theoretical framework (the context tapestry into which the research is woven). At the centre of the diagram are the anticipated steps we would normally expect: generation of a research question, collection of data to address that question, data analysis and conclusions, writing up the thesis (or argument) and presenting it for public display and critique. However,

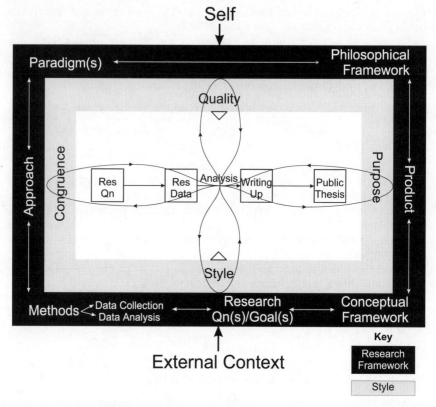

Figure 4.1 A (meta-) frame for qualitative research.

this is but the outward or observable face of research. Research needs to be embedded in a (meta-) framework comprising a congruent, coherent, dynamic matching of research goals/questions/intended product, research paradigm and its philosophical framework, the conceptual or theoretical framework which informs the research and the strategies (the general approach and the specific methods of data collection and analysis). These dimensions are analysed for the three research paradigms in Table 4.3. Interweaving between this (meta-) framework and the actions of research lie the elements of style of the research, including congruence, personal style, quality (particularly the ethical implementation of the research) and researcher's purpose. These elements of research are in fluid balance and interaction as indicated by the infinite loops.

The following extract from a doctoral thesis abstract (Titchen, 2000) illustrates beautifully such a framework in action:

> *Within a critical social science perspective, I used the distinct, but comple-*
> *mentary, traditions of phenomenological sociology and existential phenom-*
> *enology to conduct a case study of an expert in patient-centred nursing. I*
> *investigated the expert's clinical work and the experiential learning support*
> *she gave to staff nurses in a busy ward. Using action research, I also studied*
> *how I helped the expert to become a more effective facilitator of learning. I*

gathered data, over two and a half years, through participant observation, in-depth interviews, story-telling and review of documentation, and analysed them using principles developed from the three research approaches. The nature and complexity of professional craft knowledge in patient-centred nursing and in facilitating experiential learning were revealed. Theorized accounts of this knowledge are offered through two inductively derived conceptual frameworks for the helping relationships of 'skilled companionship' and 'critical companionship'. The frameworks are imbued by humanistic, phenomenological and spiritual perspectives. A critical perspective also imbues 'critical companionship'. Both use the metaphor of a companion accompanying another on a journey as a carrier of a range of theoretical ideas and symbols. I test the frameworks against the empirical research literature and ground them in rich, contextualizing data.

Personal stance – bringing self to research

One of the rich opportunities and challenges in qualitative research is bringing self into the research. In part this is the intrusion of the real-world context of the researcher (e.g. rules, resources, finances, norms, funding, space). In part it is the personal frame of reference and the lived experiences of the researcher shaping the research (for instance framing the question or setting the scope of the study). The latter notion is picked up in the following section. Several researchers in my research project on qualitative research experiences (QRP project) raised the topic of bringing self to one's research, for example:

My research question arose from my work background which is in staff development – if you like – employee development in fact, so it comes from a managerial perspective and also from a personal perspective of employees. (QRP – RP3)

Dancing on the celestial carpet

Many of us, I'm sure, have been inspired by the following quote and challenged not only to see more clearly by learning from the works of others but also to leave our own legacy for others to build on in the future.

We are dwarfs on the shoulders of giants, we can see more and further than they, not because we have keener eyesight or because we are taller than they, but because we are raised up and held aloft by their grandeur. (Master Bishop Fulbert, of Chartres Cathedral)

Building on this image I have developed a metaphor to use with my research students: dancing on the (celestial) carpet. As part of preparing the frame for their research I ask the students to construct a theoretical framework (or carpet) which, like a cognitive map or a celestial star chart, weaves together fields of knowledge (both propositional and experiential) needed to inform the research investigation. They go back in space and time and reflect on existing knowledge, understanding and questions in their given field, and map out this carpet/chart. The carpet provides a foundation for their new knowing, as a carpet woven from the tapestries of the knowledge of time, capturing and transforming the patterns and designs of knowledge, or a new vision of a star chart based on recent as well as ancient exploration of the galaxies. The students are encouraged to view their knowledge generation as not just standing on the carpet but rather dancing on it. The dancing reflects a sense of confidence in the thoroughness of the preparation of the theoretical framework, a sense of joy or excitement as the concepts and theories become integrated/ woven into the student's knowledge and a deeper understanding results, and a sense of liberation which builds on the joy and confidence as the dancer learns the power and opportunity of taking risks in exploration of self and topic. The research process involves the student's increasingly knowledgeable and rich understanding of the field, based on the experiential, personal, empirical and theoretical knowledge arising from the research. The students are creating their own new charts, which will in turn guide new explorers.

Thus the construction and use of this conceptual framework is a critical moment, both in its important role in mapping the terrain of the research and in the sense of being a catalyst for change and growth. In constructing this framework students recognize that new knowledge (derived from research projects) is generated into and within existing knowledge frameworks and builds upon existing knowledge. This knowledge is used to formulate and re-shape research questions or topics, to avoid the trap of reinventing the wheel, and to complement and inform the choice and use of the research paradigm and methods.

The framing of research questions within the philosophical and theoretical frameworks adopted by the researcher was a common theme in the interviews conducted in the QRP project. The following quote illustrates this theme:

> *Researchers need a conceptual framework for their research, otherwise they will produce acontextual ahistorical atemporal accounts . . . and be decontextualized . . . apart from producing wonderful stories you need to see the architecture. I feel that people (i.e. consumers of the research) need an architecture (structure) but they also need all the flesh (depth) and so I felt that I should frame my questions so I can take advantage of these two and I can produce a product so that it has a conceptual framework but it's also grounded in data so I can combine the oomph of the two. (QRP – RP1)*

The importance of setting the stage is powerfully illustrated by Bridgman (2000, p. 58) in her research on women in medicine. In her chapter 'Reworking – Women – Identity, Work and Power' she writes:

> *This chapter sets the stage for women, in work and in their relationships with power. It provides another thread of the context in which women find themselves (professionally and personally), when it discusses the recent his-story of the traditions of Australian society from 1880 to today, the traditions which have influenced the current meaning of our femininity. It is a his-story of the contradictions and constraints that the world has imposed/imposes upon women; a 'story' of the lives of women (including myself) who have been confronted by the maze of gender imperatives, the demand that they be 'good women'. Its purpose is to uncover the processes of becoming a woman in twentieth century Australia so that, by understanding our his-storical construction as women, we may expand our opportunities, and choose less inhibiting and stereotyped possibilities.*

What are the major fields of literature and theoretical constructs which will serve to frame your research? Table 4.4 provides some theoretical fields that can serve to frame research projects and theses.

Illuminating the phenomenon

What is the goal of research? Research seeks to illuminate the phenomenon under investigation; to increase our understanding of that phenomenon, to add to the body of knowledge about the topic or question, and to be conducted in a way that helps to bring the phenomenon to life rather than to reduce or confine it by using limited or inappropriate methods.

Thus 'illuminating the phenomenon' is a goal, a reflection of the method and the outcomes, and it describes the legacy the research leaves behind. This process is achieved through the decisions the researcher makes, the authenticity with which the chosen strategy is enacted, the congruence achieved among the various elements of the research process (as examined in the section on framing the research journey) and the way the research is communicated through writing, presentations and so on.

Choosing, phrasing and framing the research question – mapping the stellar journey

Figure 4.2 shows the research question being framed in the personal, theoretical, philosophical and methodological frameworks of the research project. Each of these frameworks interacts with the research question (or topic) as precursor or consequence. What is the goal the researcher/traveller is seeking to attain? In the planning and implementation of this journey, what are the intended directions and means of travel? What issues of feasibility need to be considered? While research needs to commence with a preliminary or working question, the actual research question can emerge almost anywhere during the course of the research. The initial question is progressively refined and developed; what it finally becomes is not grasped perhaps until the end of the research. The emergence of the research question is influenced by the researcher's approach, the research strategy, the serendipity and unexpectedness of the data or analysis findings, the ownership (by individual or group, for instance) of the project and the complexity of the topic. This is one of the freedoms of interpretive research, in particular. QRP participants describe a number of approaches to shaping the question:

> *Phrasing the question, the words chosen and the message conveyed, involves a considered use of language. If I want to emphasize a particular research approach or philosophy, if I want to consider the other senses beyond the commonly privileged verbal and visual senses – these things need to be conveyed in the research question and in the research writing. (QRP – RP12)*

> *In a way the research topic/question was an image of me (the researcher) so I wanted the idea of valuing people to be clearly present. (QRP – RP3)*

> *Framing the question was quite a challenge. I didn't know what to ask. First I had to listen to my participants talking about their experiences. Then I started*

Table 4.4 Theoretical framework dimensions (examples) (Bullock and Trombley, 1999)

Critical social science

For example any approach in social science that has a central concern with critically evaluating society for the purpose of improving it. It involves digging beneath the surface of social phenomena and questioning the assumptions on which common sense knowledge of society is based. There is an emphasis on power, inequality, exploitation and oppression, and a belief that praxis should be linked to research. Critical social scientists reject the idea that social scientists should pursue value-freedom and advocate understanding the social world from the perspective of the exploited.

Feminism

Its broad meaning is the advocacy of the rights of women. There is no single accepted definition, and feminism encompasses agitation for political and legal rights, equal opportunities, sexual autonomy, and the right of self-determination.... Feminism is a set of ideas linked to a social movement for change (a subset of critical social science).

Historicism

(Original meaning) An approach which emphasizes the uniqueness of all historical phenomena and maintains that each age should be interpreted in terms of its own ideas and principles, or negatively, that the actions of men (sic) in the past should not be explained by reference to the beliefs, motives and valuations of the historian's own epoch.

Postmodernism

A controversial term for defining the overall direction of experimental tendencies in Western arts, architecture, media, etc. since the 1950s, particularly recent developments associated with post-industrial society and cultural globalization. ... Postmodernism designates a still-amorphous body of cultural trends and directions, marked by eclecticism, pluriculturalism, and post-industrial, hi-tech, internationalist frame of reference, coupled with a sceptical view of the technical progress which nonetheless enables many of its manifestations.... To date, it remains best seen as a complex map of late twentieth century cultural expressions, social directions, fantasies and anxieties, rather than as a clear-cut aesthetic or philosophical ideology.

Poststructuralism

A set of extremely influential cultural theories, which share some of the central thematics and much of the theoretical vocabulary of structuralism, but which abandon the older structuralist aspiration to scientificity, on the ground that meaning is ultimately always indeterminate. The three key figures in this movement were Jacques Derrida, Michel Foucault (1926–1984) and Jacques Lacan (1902–1981).

Professionalization

One of the key features of the emergence of 'modern society', it has been claimed, is the transformation of many occupations into professions. This process involves the development of formal entry qualifications based upon education and examinations, the emergence of regulatory bodies with powers to admit and discipline members, and some degree of state-guaranteed monopoly rights.

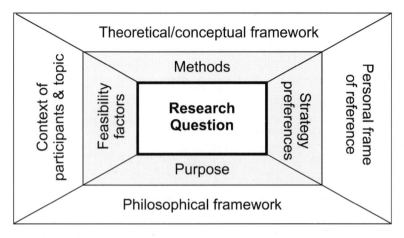

Figure 4.2 Framing research questions – frameworks dimensions (© Higgs 1998).

> *to develop understanding of … {the phenomenon} and I was able to derive some questions. (QRP – RP7)*

> *I start with writing down what I'm thinking and what I want to achieve, and I have a brainstorm with myself on paper and I have to have a period of cogitation and then I usually talk it through with a couple of people. Then I try out a few questions and see if I can develop them, see if I can find a way of writing a brief resume of what I'm after and it takes me a long time but I keep refining that and trying it out again till I get something that I think is OK and I'll probably keep changing it. (QRP – RP6)*

Writing the research

Lee (1998, p. 122) draws attention to the profoundly textual nature of research. She argues that:

> *… there is a complex relationship between knowledge and language, between coming to know and coming to write, between matters integral to the doing of a PhD such as research design, method and analysis, and the production of the thesis text. And there is a complex relationship between the production of knowledge through the practices of writing, and subjectivity, the production of a particular kind of knower/writer. Yet these relationships are often poorly understood, at least in terms of the ways research is commonly conceptualized.… There has been little attention paid to the question of writing, that central, difficult and often trauma-ridden activity of the production of the doctoral thesis.*

Writing is a powerful tool for coming to know, for learning to write as well as for interpreting the data and illuminating the research process and product. In a text on *Writing Qualitative Research* (Higgs, 1998), various authors provide chapters discussing factors relating to matching the writing to the phenomenon and/or the research method – for example, 'Constructing a narrative' (Goodfellow, 1998), 'Language and style in phenomenological research' (Smith, 1998), 'Describing the phenomenon'

(Crotty, 1998b) and 'Adopting a phenomenological philosophy to research and writing' (Lawler, 1998). A QRP researcher describes the writing style adopted:

> *In telling these stories here I am seeking to give voice to the storytellers and also to the players in their stories: students, novice researchers, opponents, sceptics and support people – all of them shape the central arguments being presented. I think that having a vision of how to deal with these critical moments involves understanding that research and decisions about research are encapsulated within the character and identity of cultures, the understandings and limitations inherent in language and the expectations and notions associated with quality and scholarship. (QRP – RP10)*

Illuminating the phenomenon, answering the question – choosing an appropriate method

A key issue researchers face is deciding whether, when and how to mix research paradigms and approaches. For those who consider that differences in research approaches are primarily technical, the 'mixing and matching' of research methods is considered acceptable (Goodwin and Goodwin, 1984). If differences in paradigms are considered to be primarily epistemological (i.e. different ways of knowing about phenomena) then it is argued that such mixing violates the philosophical intent and purposes of each paradigm (Leininger, 1994). This issue needs to be considered by researchers when formulating their research questions and selecting their research framework. Brew (1998) argues in favour of moving beyond paradigm boundaries. She explores the question: 'How can we invent new methodologies for research and new forms of expression while at the same time being academically rigorous and respectable?'. Part of the answer to this question has already been addressed in this chapter in terms of understanding the methodology and learning to live it authentically, challenging the traditional constraints and standards, and re-framing what it means to be rigorous against standards more suitable to the chosen research strategy.

The term 'illuminating the phenomenon' was chosen to contain a notion of enhancing rather than damaging the phenomenon as well as seeking to understand it. This not only requires an appropriate choice of method which respects and allows rich engagement with the phenomenon; it also requires authenticity by the researcher(s) in the mode of this engagement. Such authenticity requires a depth of understanding of the research paradigm and its philosophy, heightened awareness by researchers of their own as well as participants' experiences and perceptions of the research process, and a clear understanding of how the research process needs to be implemented to achieve this authenticity. There is a close relationship here between ethics and authenticity. Research ethics is not limited to a rather clinical view of 'doing no harm'; it also needs to be reflected in the closeness of fit (the congruence) between the researcher's espoused theory/philosophy and the theory or research strategy in action, hence authenticity.

Exemplar

In the following extract from a thesis abstract (Bridgman, 2000) we see a vivid example of a thesis which richly illuminated the phenomenon under investigation; 'Rhythms of awakening: Re-membering the her-story and mythology of women in medicine':

> This thesis is based on the stories of the lived experience of two groups of women, the first was a group of women healers working in many areas of medicine, and the second, a group of academic women. Their stories have been woven into a his-storical, mythological and theoretical context.
>
> To add depth to the story I have critiqued both science and scientific medicine, while offering more holistic alternatives as part of this process. Mainstream medicine is firmly rooted in the positivist paradigm but in this thesis I am using a multi-method approach, namely feminist research, cooperative inquiry and narrative, all of which are part of the post-positivist discourse.
>
> The thesis has been constructed with a series of stories to acknowledge the uniqueness of each individual's experience. While each experience is valid in itself, at some level it also forms part of the consciousness of all humanity. The narrative construction of experience is an innate process common to all cultures. Humans seek to organize their experiences into meaningful unities and the way we do this is to use story. These stories therefore provide the threads that weave this thesis together and are congruent with both the process of the making of meaning in our lives, and with our journeys towards healing.
>
> The research is embedded in both a socialist feminist framework and that of depth psychology/mythology. It is based on feminist research methods and cooperative inquiry methodology and uses narrative for the recounting of the experience. My position as a woman, a healer and an eco-feminist giving it its flavour and colour. It is also a heuristic inquiry that offers constructive critique using reflexive learning and explores the richness of difference in philosophies of healing and the experience of transformation.

Conversing with peers and sages

In the QRP research project (Higgs and Radovich, 1999) we asked researchers conducting interpretive and critical paradigm research about the factors which facilitated positive and quality research outcomes in interpretive and critical paradigm research. Their responses included:

- the capacity and supportiveness of research supervisors/mentors
- the supportiveness of the research environment
- the capacity of researchers to persevere in the face of inevitable difficulties encountered during qualitative research
- the researcher's experience in performing qualitative research – this experience was a matter of quality of understanding and assurance rather than quantity (e.g. volume or duration) of research implemented
- peer interaction and critical companionship
- an understanding of the impact of context, theoretical frameworks and personal frames of reference on research design and implementation.

Three critical elements track across these factors: education, support and interaction. These activities may well be described as conversing with peers and sages. As researchers we learn much from our mentors who provide inspiration, insights and the benefit of their experience, and we learn much from our peers who are often grappling with the same dilemmas and confusions we are facing. Both these factors enhance the supportiveness of the environment for what can often be a long and challenging research journey. For the researcher or research student who is working largely alone, the lack of these supports is often strongly felt.

Finally, conversing with peers and sages functions as a reminder to send our work out for public scrutiny, so that our findings, tested by the field, can become part of the knowledge of that field. Such testing and scrutiny, however, is best not all left to the end. The wise researcher, student and supervisor know the value of seeking input from peers (receiving challenging, sometimes unexpected questions which make us sit back and re-think our strategy and rationale) and from sages (whose depth of knowledge of the topic, related or even tangential fields, or methodology raises our capacity to dance on richer carpets and critically appraise or defend our work).

Conclusion

Charting standpoints in qualitative research has been described as a journey, like space and time travelling, in which research travellers learn to chart their way by constructing a framework which, deeply understood, imbues their actions with authenticity, confidence, direction and purpose. While the times of confusion, of being lost in space and time, may be just the void needed to spark inspiration, imagination and a strong sense of purpose, other supportive contexts like education and peer appraisal provide the enthusiasm or re-energizing which is vital in the (often) long haul or critical pressure moments of research.

[1] This and other similar quotes in this chapter are derived from a narrative inquiry project I am conducting, titled Qualitative Research Project (QRP), dealing with the experiences of qualitative researchers working in tertiary education contexts. RP1 refers to Research Participant 1 (etc.) in this study. A preliminary report of this study appears in Higgs and Radovich (1999).

References

Barnett, R. (1990) *The Idea of Higher Education*. Buckingham: The Society for Research into Higher Education and Open University Press.

Beeston, S. and Higgs, J. (2001) Professional practice: artistry and connoisseurship. In *Practice Knowledge and Expertise in the Health Professions* (J. Higgs and A. Titchen, eds), pp. 108–117. Oxford: Butterworth-Heinemann.

Benner, P. (1984) *From Novice to Expert: Excellence and Power in Clinical Nursing Practice*. London: Addison-Wesley.

Benner, P. and Wrubel, J. (1989) *The Primacy of Caring: Stress and Coping in Health and Illness*. Wokingham: Addison-Wesley.

Benner, P., Tanner, C. and Chesla, C. (1996) *Expertise in Nursing Practice: Caring, Clinical Judgement and Ethics*. New York: Springer Publishing.

Berger, P. and Luckmann, T. (1985) *The Social Construction of Reality*. Harmondsworth: Penguin.

Berlin, I. (1979) *Against the Current: Essays in the History of Ideas* (H. Hardy, ed.). London: Hogarth Press.

Bogdan, R. C. and Bilken, S. K. (1992) *Qualitative Research for Education: An Introduction to Theory and Methods*, 2nd edn. Boston: Allyn and Bacon.

Brew, A. (1998) Moving beyond paradigm boundaries. In *Writing Qualitative Research* (J. Higgs, ed.), pp. 29–46. Sydney: Hampden Press.

Bridgman, K. E. (2000) Rhythms of awakening: re-membering the her-story and mythology of women in medicine. PhD thesis, University of Western Sydney, Hawkesbury, NSW, Australia.

Brown, S. and McIntyre, D. (1993) *Making Sense of Teaching*. Milton Keynes: Open University Press.

Bullock, A. and Trombley, S. (1999) *The New Fontana Dictionary of Modern Thought*, 3rd edn. London: Harper Collins.

Burnard, P. (1992) *Writing for Health Professionals: A Manual for Writers*. London: Chapman and Hall.

Candy, P. C. (1991) *Self-Direction for Lifelong Learning*. San Francisco: Jossey-Bass.

Crotty, M. (1998a) *The Foundations of Social Research: Meaning and Perspective in the Research Process*. St Leonards: Allen and Unwin.

Crotty, M. (1998b) Describing the phenomenon. In *Writing Qualitative Research* (J. Higgs, ed.), pp. 205–216. Sydney: Hampden Press.

Denzin, N. K. and Lincoln, Y. S. (eds) (1994) *Handbook of Qualitative Research*. Thousand Oaks: Sage.

Domholdt, E. (1993) *Physical Therapy Research: Principles and Applications*. Philadelphia: W. B. Saunders.

Edwards, H. (1997) Clinical teaching: an exploration in three health professions. PhD thesis, University of Melbourne, Australia.

Eisner, E. (1985) *The Art of Educational Evaluation: A Personal View*. London: The Falmer Press.

Eraut, M. (1985) Knowledge creation and knowledge use in professional contexts. *Studies in Higher Education*, **10**(2), 117–133.

Fetterman D. (1988) *Qualitative Approaches to Evaluation: The Silent Scientific Revolution*. New York: Praeger.

Fish, D. (1998) *Appreciating Practice in the Caring Professions: Refocusing Professional Development and Practitioner Research*. Oxford: Butterworth-Heinemann.

Flew, A. (ed.) (1984) *A Dictionary of Philosophy*, 2nd edn. London: Pan.

French, S. (1993) *Practical Research: A Guide for Therapists*. Oxford: Butterworth-Heinemann.

Gadamer, H.-G. (1975) Hermeneutics and social science. *Cultural Hermeneutics*, **2**, 307–316.

Goodfellow, J. (1998) Constructing a narrative. In *Writing Qualitative Research* (J. Higgs, ed.), pp. 175–188. Sydney: Hampden Press.

Goodwin, L. D. and Goodwin, W. L. (1984) Qualitative vs quantitative research or qualitative *and* quantitative research? *Nursing Research*, **33**, 378–380.

Guba, E. (1978) *Towards a Methodology of Naturalistic Inquiry in Educational Evaluation: Monograph 8*. Los Angeles: UCLA Centre for the Study of Evaluation.

Habermas, J. (1972) *Knowledge and Human Interests*. London: Heinemann.

Heidegger, M. (1962) *Being and Time*. New York: Harper and Row.

Higgs, J. (1998) Structuring qualitative research theses. In *Writing Qualitative Research* (J. Higgs, ed.), pp. 137–150. Sydney: Hampden Press.

Higgs, J. and Radovich, S. (1999) Narratives on Qualitative Research. *AQR '99 International Conference on Issues of Rigour in Qualitative Research*, 8–10 July 1999, Melbourne, Australia.

Higgs, J. and Titchen, A. (1995) The nature, generation and verification of knowledge. *Physiotherapy*, **81**(9), 521–530.

Higgs, J. and Titchen, A. (1998) Research and knowledge. *Physiotherapy*, **84**(2), 72–80.

Higgs, J. and Titchen, A. (eds) (2001) *Practice Knowledge and Expertise in the Health Professions*. Oxford: Butterworth-Heinemann.

Higgs, J., Maxwell, I., Fredericks, I. and Spence L. (2001a) Developing creative arts expertise. In *Professional Practice in Health, Education and the Creative Arts* (J. Higgs and A. Titchen, eds), pp. 238–250. Oxford: Blackwell Science.

Higgs, J., Titchen, A. and Neville, V. (2001b) Professional practice and knowledge. In *Practice Knowledge and Expertise in the Health Professions* (J. Higgs and A. Titchen, eds), pp. 3–9. Oxford: Butterworth-Heinemann.

Howe, K. R. (1985) Two dogmas of educational research. *Educational Researcher*, **October**, 10–18.

Howe, K. R. (1988) Against the quantitative–qualitative incompatibility thesis. *Educational Researcher*, **November**, 10–16.

Lawler, J. (1998) Adopting a phenomenological philosophy to research and writing. In *Writing Qualitative Research* (J. Higgs, ed.), pp. 47–58. Sydney: Hampden Press.

Lee, A. (1998) Doctoral research as writing. In *Writing Qualitative Research* (J. Higgs, ed.), pp. 121–134. Sydney: Hampden Press.

Leininger, M. M. (1994) Evaluation criteria and critique of qualitative research studies. In *Critical Issues in Qualitative Research Methods* (J. M. Morse, ed.), pp. 95–115. Thousand Oaks: Sage.

Leonard, V. A. (1989) A Heideggerian phenomenologic perspective on the concept of the person. *Advances in Nursing Science*, **11**, 40–55.

Lincoln, Y. S. and Guba, E. (1985) *Naturalistic Inquiry*. Newbury Park: Sage.

MacLeod, M. (1990) Experience in everyday nursing practice: a study of 'experienced' ward sisters. PhD thesis, University of Edinburgh, Edinburgh, Scotland, UK.

McCarthy, E. D. (1996) *Knowledge As Culture: The New Sociology of Knowledge*. London: Routledge and Kegan Paul.

Merleau-Ponty, M. (1956) What is phenomenology? *Cross Currents*, **16**, 59–70.

Moore, T. W. (1982) *Philosophy of Education: An Introduction*. London: Routledge and Kegan Paul.

Parlett, M. and Hamilton, D. (1972) *Evaluation as Illumination: A New Approach to the Study of Innovatory Programs*. Occasional Paper No. 9., Centre for Research in the Educational Sciences, University of Edinburgh, Edinburgh, Scotland, UK.

Powers, B. A. and Knapp, T. R. (1995) *A Dictionary of Nursing Theory and Research*, 2nd edn. Thousand Oaks: Sage.

Rabinow, P. and Sullivan, M. (1979) *Interpretive Social Science*. Berkeley: University of California Press.

Rothwell, R. (1995) Science and non-experimental paradigms, history and philosophy of scientific methodology. In *1997 Program Manual* (R. Rothwell, ed.). Faculty of Health Sciences, The University of Sydney, NSW, Australia.

Schön, D. A. (1987) *Educating the Reflective Practitioner: Towards a New Design for Teaching and Learning in Professions*. San Francisco: Jossey-Bass.

Smith, D. (1998) Language and style in phenomenological research. In *Writing Qualitative Research* (J. Higgs, ed.), pp. 189–195. Sydney: Hampden Press.

Smith, J. K. (1983) Quantitative versus qualitative research: An attempt to clarify the issue. *Educational Researcher*, 12, 6–13.

Smith, J. K. and Heshusius, L. (1986) Closing down the conversation: end of the quantitative–qualitative debate among educational inquirers. *Educational Researcher*, **January**, 4–12.

Tesch, R. (1992) *Qualitative Research: Analysis Types and Software Tools*. London: Falmer Press.

Thorne, S. (1997) The art and science of critiquing qualitative research. In *Completing a Qualitative Project: Details and Dialogue* (J. M. Morse, ed.), pp. 117–132. Thousand Oaks: Sage.

Titchen, A. (2000) *Professional Craft Knowledge in Patient-Centred Nursing and the Facilitation of its Development*. DPhil thesis, University of Oxford, Oxford, UK. Oxford: Ashdale Press.

Titchen, A. and Higgs, J. (2001) Towards professional artistry and creativity in practice. In *Professional Practice in Health, Education and the Creative Arts* (J. Higgs and A. Titchen, eds), pp. 271–290. Oxford: Blackwell Science.

Usher, R. (1996) A critique of the neglected epistemological assumptions of educational research. In *Understanding Educational Research* (D. Scott and R. Usher, eds), pp. 9–32. London: Routledge and Kegan Paul.

5

Re-authoring self:[1] knowing as being

Hilary Byrne-Armstrong

At the time of editing this book I completed (successfully, I am pleased to say!) a PhD thesis (Byrne-Armstrong, 1999). It would be difficult not to think that the process of completing arguably the biggest academic project a student undertakes and having the idea for this book were not in some way connected. The early ideas for this book emerged out of a retreat in which 30 people gathered for three days to begin to plan and write a book that will soon be published. In my talking and gossiping with academics from many disciplines about their experiences of undergoing the task in which I was immersed, I was told many tales that eased what were, at the time, my very private agonies. In fact, not only did these conversations relieve me of a crisis I was secretly having, they also influenced the project in a significant way. No longer did I feel the necessity to separate my life and my research. In fact, I saw how they could be framed as one and the same process.

For a start, if I had not experienced dilemmas and critical moments in my teaching and research, I would not have been interested enough to sustain the energy that it takes to complete a PhD. Furthermore, I perhaps did not need to hide the fact that what I started out to do was no longer valid intellectually for me. You see, (un)fortunately, the reading and researching I did as a result of undertaking the project changed and shifted it both paradigmatically and methodologically. I began to see this change not as a problem but as a strength; not as an issue separate to the research but as the research itself; not as something separate from the researcher but as the learning of the researcher herself; epistemology as ontology.

In this chapter I trace the process of 'constructing the thesis I did', a very different thesis to the one I set out to produce, and show how, in this process, I re-authored myself. I changed from a self that researched others' learning transitions to one that recognized mine as inextricably woven with these others; from one that researched collaboratively to one that moved away from these methods on the grounds of ethics (see Chapter 8). But most significantly, a thesis emerged that demonstrates that researching, my knowledge production and practice are not separable; that the play between theory, practice and life keeps the material alive and embodied. This play is also messy, chaotic and contingent. Writing a thesis that was reflexive and that demonstrated itself was therefore a challenge. Like the thesis this chapter necessarily will fall short of its aims, but, like the thesis, it does this with acknowledgment that there is always a fine line, an 'ironic tension', when practising reflexivity in the context of academic practice. It is this tension and my negotiation through it that enabled the re-authoring of self, and it is this story that makes up this chapter.

My thesis documented the development of a narrative epistemology in pedagogy, heralding a progressive shift away from individualistic accounts of conflicts and dilemmas in learning as being primarily embedded in psychological spaces, to a recognition of the importance of the social space: the cultural discourses that shape our everyday activity and interactions. Conflict, then, is not simply a consequence of difference arising from personality, or other psychological factors, but a consequence of prevailing cultural narratives that instruct/construct us into the identities we are.

My initial questions/conflicts emerged as a student and teacher within a particular tradition of radical education. I term this in the thesis, the 'local radical pedagogy'. I became concerned with the social forms within this tradition that constructed 'right' and 'wrong' models of learning, 'true' and 'false' consciousness, reduced the complexity of human beings and their worlds to quadrant models of learning styles and personality profile categories, and preached prescriptions for reflective self-styling practices. My search was to deconstruct (through my own practice) some of these so-called radical teaching practices; to find out for myself how much they perpetuate the very forms of exploitation and subjugation that they purport to challenge. I was not doing this within the politics of the pointing finger; if anywhere, the finger gestured in my direction, as someone who at times was too uncritical about the truth of stories informing my practice.

The exploration of a range of teaching and learning practices centred around the development of a 'narrative epistemology'; that is, a way of knowing that holds the social space open for multi-storied narratives, and recognizes the politics of difference between narratives. The more I became familiar with my topic, the more dilemmas I found as I came to construct a thesis. As I was basing my work in feminist and poststructuralist epistemologies, it was important for me to be reflexive, to walk my talk(s), and talk my walk(s)! How to do this within the confines of the conventions of a thesis was the question. As an academic, I was all too aware that although many people begin their research journey with dreams of producing a radically different thesis, most people recognize when it comes to the crunch that to do it well, with rigour, is actually more difficult and more time consuming than to write a traditional thesis. I therefore had set out to write a traditional thesis. However, as my learning changed, and the self that I was becoming disturbed my initial epistemology, I found myself unable to consider this option, in fact unable to contemplate writing in any other way than I did. Thus, as well as being a document that expounds a narrative epistemology, the thesis is written as a demonstration of the thinking and exploring that I did in my elaboration of this epistemology as I recreated myself as a teacher and learner. In other words, in participating in this research, rather than gaining a body of knowledge, I have tested assumptions that I have about the world I inhabit, discarded some, modified others and recreated my subjectivity.

The main theorist I drew on was Foucault (1983),[2] who wrote that there were three types of struggle:

- the struggle against forms of exploitation (ethnic, social and religious)
- the struggle against forms of exploitation that separate individuals from what they produce (economic)
- the struggle that ties the individual to her/himself and submits her/him to others in this way (forms of subjection, subjectivity and submission).

Education is implicated in all of these forms of exploitation. That is obvious in mainstream education. In radical/experiential forms of education it is less obvious and more subtle, but nevertheless present. But as well as being implicated in exploitation and oppression, education also promotes agency and autonomy (as anyone who has written a research thesis will know!). The tension inherent in this paradox is central to my project and its outcomes, and central to my learning and changing subjectivity in the production of my thesis. My aim was to unpack this tension and demonstrate that the dance inherent in this paradox is the heart, the stuff to be worked with as a reconstructionist teacher (Gore, 1993). My imperative, therefore, was to make this dance (I called it an ironic tension) central to the thesis.

Knowing and being dilemmas

This imperative, in the context of thesis construction and presentation, presented several dilemmas. I proposed that the activity of deconstructing the ironic tension opens the space for people to conform or resist and therefore acquire some agency and autonomy in the face of subjugating discourses. Furthermore, deconstructing the complexities of our lives makes the material base of knowledge visible, thus showing that the social forms that we dream up as human beings are historical, contingent, multiple and partial, making visible the fissures through which resistance and agency can occur. And, as the different stories that shape our lives are 'sung-up', we hear a chorus of voices rather than just one or two voices. Allowing this cacophony to sing is, I proposed, an ethical basis of practice, and a position of potential conflict and tension. My dilemma was how to make this position visible within the constraints of the academic (or social) form called a PhD thesis and to produce an acceptable thesis. One of the main features of the narrative epistemology I was proposing is verisimilitude: 'lifelikeness'. Lifelikeness began with the use of my own teaching/learning practices as the data for exploration. But constructing a thesis that demonstrated verisimilitude required more than this; it required that the research methods be compatible with the pedagogy. In other words, the research methods that I used in the thesis had to be the same as those I used in my learning and teaching. In these loops of (self) reflexive practice, the risk of self-delusion was high. My response was to position myself in an ironic tension, a sort of detached engagement. My thesis, while academically sound (detached), had also to embody verisimilitude (engaged).

The production of knowledge is not a clear and systematic process; it is whimsical and unpredictable. This in itself is a challenge for thesis writing. Then there is the aspect of the unknown reader. I interwove knowledge generated from the community of scholars I was reading (commonly called 'theory') with knowledge generated by the community of scholars who were my students (commonly called 'practice'). However, the reader is also present as another (unknown) participant in the process. His/her reading of the thesis generated knowledge (as well as assessment). How could I write a thesis that kept the reader engaged as an active participant (recognizing I had little control if I did not keep to traditional forms), and successfully complete the task?

Finally, a major learning outcome of the thesis (and my self re-authoring) was coming to the realization of the importance of holding the discursive space open. An open conversational space allows contradictions, inconsistencies, anomalies and conflicts to be visible, but it presents a dilemma when writing a thesis. A thesis is traditionally one in which these things are sanitized out, where the discursive space is gradually and systematically closed down in the name of results and conclusions. My dilemma was to manifest the dream of writing a thesis in which the discursive space was kept open and free floating, and still maintain an integrity as a piece of academic writing.

Knowing and being responses

1. Feminism

The feminist stance of the thesis is reflected throughout. As a feminist researcher, I was aware that not only was I doing research with women, but also the research was feminist in other ways (Horsfall, 1997).

I positioned myself initially at an intersection of radical experiential education, cultural feminism and interpretive traditions, to fit within the broad endeavour of my lifework. This positioning reflects cultural feminism in that it 'concretely and analytically locate[d] the product of the ... labour process within a concrete analysis of the process of production itself' (Stanley, 1990, p. 12). Through engagement with work my voice had been growing in clarity (and loudness). However, in using the personal pronoun for thesis writing rather than the 'normal' dominant, abstract, patriarchal voice of academic culture, I knew I was taking a risk of being criticized for swimming around in untheorized raw data (i.e. subjectivity), '[a] kind of pre-theoretical chaos' (see Stanley, 1990, p. 42) that could be considered unscientific and devoid of theoretical implications. This criticism, of course, assumes that there is such a thing as 'raw' data. From the feminist positioning I was taking there is no such thing. Experience is never raw, it is always constitutive of a 'first order' theorizing (Stanley, 1990, p. 42), an interpretation and a narrative embedded in history and culture. This position reflects the 'feminist insistence on the determined conjoining of the dichotomies, a refusal to accept that such divisions exist within a world of experience' (Stanley, 1990, p. 11). Knowledge is material and embodied. The process of knowledge construction that is called a thesis was my lived experience.

Feminists write extensively of the political processes of phallocentric discourse that separate the researcher from the researched (see Nicholson, 1990; Stanley, 1990; Kreiger, 1991; Reinharz, 1992). My thesis 'draws the process of knowledge production, in researching and theory, into its *product* in the shape of written accounts of it' (Stanley, 1990, p. 4). It historically traced the narratives of my lived experience as I lived, and showed the production of knowledge that led me to re-author these stories and my lifework.

I also found myself fully recognizing the enormous courage, power and strength of those mothers who had held the space open for me to construct and write a thesis that embodied my gender and socialization. There is still a slippery boundary between what is my voice and these voices of others, the mothers, those wise women before me whose work contributed to my voice in the thesis (and the fathers whose vision for a better world contributed to their enterprise). And, as I was engaged in the patriarchal project of writing a thesis, I used at times a voice that engaged in contest and argumentation. I also struggled with a task (impossible?) to find a voice that disengaged from contestation; a voice and language that was not 'from the sameness' of which Irigaray (1980) spoke. In the broader scheme of things, both/all these voices, heard in their difference, can and do contribute to all lives in the shadow of the powerful discourses that shape docile bodies in the name of capitalism, humanism and patriarchy (Foucault, 1977). For my voice to emerge, I returned to the wisdom of the mothers and to my version of the central tenets of feminist scholarship. Out of this I hoped that a voice would emerge that spoke 'from herself' with the purpose of speaking to others to make visible the web that connects, not in a sentimental sense but in a pragmatic sense. I therefore justified my choice of writing style as personal, narrative and at times poetic.

The positioning of the author self-reflexively within a text is pivotal to the cultural feminist project of which I am a part. Firstly, as mentioned above, the first person voice was used. Secondly, this positioning makes transparent the actual process of knowledge production and the subjectivities and identities that constituted my voice as this knowledge was produced. This makes it a feminist thesis in the sense of walking the path of knowledge construction while reflecting on my construction of it. Thirdly, it is presented as a narrative and, in this sense, is reflexive: it is a demonstration of what it is about.

Feminism gave me a voice to speak the dilemmas I encountered as a feminist teacher and researcher. 'The feminist teacher is a kind of ... in fact ... a strange creature – neither father or mother' (Gore, 1993, p. 69). The duty of care that was regarded as central to early feminist ethics and moral views informed this work and also provided one of its central dilemmas. This dilemma I identified as a dichotomy in (my construction of) teaching. On one hand there is the 'authority' of a more masculine perspective (the universal ethic of justice and rights built on objectivity, detachment and individual autonomy), and on the other there is the 'duty of care' (a feminist perspective based on intersubjectivity, nurturance, particularity and emotion). Some would say that the tension between these two roles/positions is not new (Browning Cole and Coultrap-McQuin, 1992), but my personal experience of it began me on this journey. Now, this tension is still present, vivid, a disturbance, and at times even fun!

2. Phenomenological hermeneutics

Early in the research I employed a hermeneutic method (what Polkinghorne (1983) termed 'phenomenological hermeneutics'). In other words, I reflected on the utterances and descriptions of a series of pedagogic events, to interpret them with the assumption that I could detach myself from my socialization (what is known as phenomenological 'bracketing'), the ability to stand back, reflect and observe things in order to discover their essence (Sass, 1990). This practice is used to discover the nature of the original experience (the essence) without the strictures of language, and is thus embedded in the assumption that experience, language and social practices can be separated (Polkinghorne, 1988). The early phenomenologists considered this so-called ability we have to suspend our presuppositions as the fundamental mode that makes meaning of human existence. It alludes to the transcendental subject of humanism: the subject beyond culture and history, beyond gender and socialization.

3. Social action: crises of knowing and being

My doubts about this proposition came from a series of pragmatic experiences in contemplative communities. Certainly reflective and meditative knowing gave people meaning in their lives, but it did not seem to help their relationships or ability to cooperate as human beings. I became 'politicized', and was engaged in ten years of social action. I travelled extensively as part of a worldwide project[3] aimed at working with social issues. In large, international, cross-cultural residentials, 200 people struggled together to understand violence, oppression and ways of understanding difference. These residentials became theatres for airing the disabling aspects of discourses of racism, ethnicity, homophobia and sexism and our collective and often internalized fears and hatreds. People shared their stories and experiences, struggled with conflict, difference and marginalization. Through these stories, I came to know that I was constructed by a social milieu; my voice was one of a white, educated middleclass academic woman, and this positioning marked me as privileged. I also lived in the shadow of powerful discourses, which shaped me as 'other'. But the degree of 'otherness' is not defined or static. In many contexts I am privileged over my colleagues and friends who are differently coloured and classed, or have other than mainstream sexual preferences. I have many stories from this time:

- I have been witness to stories of childhood sexual abuse and violence against women (especially women in 'third world' countries) and have worked in communities with women to change these disabling discourses.
- I have protested at stories of violence against people who choose other than mainstream sexuality, such as a report of a woman being flown back to the USA in a military aircraft in handcuffs and leg irons for being lesbian in the armed forces. Lesbians and gays demanded that I look at the privilege of my 'invisibility' as a white middleclass heterosexual woman. I have marched for gay and lesbian rights, and given my services to the gay community to work with those identified as people with AIDS.

- I have been yelled at in anger as a representative of a colonizing white race when I said, 'I feel hopeless, I have tried everything that I know; whatever I say or do is never enough'. The reply, 'Good, you feel despair; now you begin to know what it is like to be black in this country [USA]. Perhaps there is the first glimmer of empathy; now perhaps we can begin to talk'.

Through these experiences I came to recognize that the interpretations that I produced through reflection were more to do with my (often distorted) self-narrative than with some hidden meaning. And this recognition carried some irony, because in acknowledging the connection I was implying the feminist view I already ascribed to, in which there is no separation between the knower and known. The irony was obvious, but feminism and the process of phenomenological reduction (as I had produced it) were inadequate in the light of these experiences. This was a critical moment. My experiences in the world were at odds with my knowing, and this dilemma led me to change the epistemological position of the project. Suddenly I had decentred myself; it was now risky business to depend on my own abilities to reflect. I needed interactions with others, others whose world was at odds with mine, whose existence clashed at the edges of my awareness and dragged me into unknown and at times frightening, but always exhilarating, territories of knowledge.

At around the same time I was teaching a first-year undergraduate subject (in critical pedagogies)[4] and collecting the initial data for my thesis. A final-year student was assisting me. She was undertaking an action research project[5] and we acted as co-researchers to gather material for her project and the thesis. My co-researcher had asked the students if they would join with her to explore and explicate what she termed 'transformational learning' (Gebbie, 1994), characterized by a developmental movement in learners of three stages from dualism to relativism and, finally, contextual relativism (Salner, 1986). Our interest at the time was to trace the role of reflexivity in these stages and to follow the way in which students developed this ability. My co-researcher collected data in a variety of ways. There were sessions that were taped and transcribed, our research journals, a learning group that my co-researcher formed, and conversations.

As the project progressed, the disturbances, the struggles, the conflicts and the lack of response by (some) students to invitations to become autonomous learners formed the critical moments which were to become transformative to my learning. It became obvious to me that learning stages or reflexivity were not enough to explain the struggles students had with radical/experiential learning, or the sense of failure that I felt as an educator within it. The more I considered this position, the more I became aware of the inadequacies of (my) individualistic epistemology. For example, in groups, who/what was listened to had more to do with who spoke (and their position) than whether they were reflexive learners. My experience in the social action community served to reinforce this perception, and the two together provided the powerful launching pad for me to explore the connections between power and knowledge, the poststructuralist critique that is still missing from much radical/experiential/systems learning and writings.

4. Poststructuralism

The power and constitutive force of language and discourse began to dawn on me along with the decentring of self. The notion of the death of the author (the poststructuralist turn) opened the door to seeing the students as constituted subjects within the educational discourse. Whether in radical experiential education or in mainstream classroom practice, this discourse was still shaping our lives. The poststructuralist stance added an important dimension, the connection between power and knowledge, which had been my lived experience in the social action in which I had been involved. This stance meant a redesign of the writing and presentation of the thesis. To walk the talk(s) and talk the walk(s) of a poststructuralist thesis, I had to produce multiple interpretations. To include history and temporality I had to introduce narratives. To maintain the ironic tension I had to find other languages, such as metaphor. These stances all had to be justified.

Foucault contrasts 'real places ... which are ... messy, ill constructed and jumbled' (1986, p. 25) with the 'fundamentally unreal spaces' (Utopias) which exhibit society in a 'perfect ... meticulous' singular arrangement. The former he called 'Heterotopias'. In using a combination of the early methodology of hermeneutics, and to show the movement into the narrative form through a form of discourse analysis, I set out to demonstrate in the thesis a Heterotopia, a representation of the messy, unstructured and chaotic process that constitutes any lived learning/research/knowledge production and pedagogy. Foucault's theories provided me with the underpinnings to demonstrate what the thesis proposed: that when multiple interpretations are exposed, people begin to see the cracks and fissures in what otherwise looks like fixed and absolute truth. As a result, I arranged the research as a series of narratives with multiple interpretations which travel in a 'higgledy-piggledy' fashion in and out of theory building and theory tearing down, of trying new things, momentary passions, excitements, reflection, slumps, conversations, journal-keeping and conflicts. Because of the task at hand, I put these episodes in a more orderly fashion than actually occurred in my research and learning, but I tried to retain some of the chaos and spontaneous moments.

I aimed to demonstrate discursive openness, to illustrate the power of social life (or the habitus)[6] to direct our stories/interpretations. The assumption was that social life is an external 'space', lived by us as we take up subject positions which are constantly moving within relationships of power, delineating each other, creating a geography of space and imagination, or what Foucault (1986) called 'fields of action'. Foucault (1986, p. 14) said that our stories/interpretations have:

> ... *milieux, immediate locales, provocative emplacements which effect thought and action. The historical imagination is never completely spaceless ... it is always time and history that provide the primary variable containers in these geographies ... an already made geography sets the stage, while the willful making of history dictates the action and defines the story line.*

The research narratives were the containers that I created in order for time and history to dictate a story line/interpretation. They were arranged as discrete narratives shaped around a plot (theme) that followed certain educational themes and their philosophical underpinnings. They represent the play with the postmodern, me walking the talk and talking the walk of the thesis: that the pedagogy of the argument is the pedagogy being argued for (Gore, 1993). They traced the encounters with truth/self/power in the classroom that led me to occupy the theoretical position of the thesis and to develop and practise a narrative epistemology.

These encounters, my co-researcher's findings, further conversations with students, and my reflections over time provided the final material. Each narrative included an encounter, different theoretical views of it, different interpretations using discourse analysis, and reconfigured practices in the light of this interpretation. I employed the following metaphors to keep the central motif of ironic tension alive and structure the material:

- '*singing-up*'[7] to evoke the poststructuralist view that the ways we talk and imagine ourselves and the taken-for-granted social practices and language games that we engage in every moment are actions that constitute reality;
- '*dead-certainties*',[8] a play on words and a metaphor to gesture towards the ironic tension in modernism/postmodernism debates. The '*dead-certainties*' were the events/exercises and theories in the thesis that began each narrative. They were not examples of practices/knowledges that were bad, or outmoded. The term was chosen to throw into sharp relief the paradoxes, dilemmas and ironies that occur in any practice/ knowledge;
- '*local-knowledge*'[9] to gesture towards the notion of local, concrete and embodied knowledge production. In producing knowledge there will always be forms of resistance, actions that emerge as more comprehensive understandings are exposed of the behaviour of individuals in relations to the subjectifying practices of our culture. The local-knowledges represent the discourse analyses of the thesis that exposed these resistances;
- '*thick-descriptions*' (Geertz, 1983, pp. 89–90) to imagine the richness of realities/stories/knowledges/truths when there is discursive openness. In the thesis, the thick descriptions represent my reconfigured practices in the light of my learning. Whether this learning is a theory story or a practice story, the thick descriptions expand the available knowledges through several examples, thus giving the reader an opportunity to dialogue with the text in several ways.

I used this structure not to suggest progression towards something better/ truthful/more correct, but to gesture towards a narrative epistemology. In other words, I added to and expanded my praxis over time, rather than refining it to a single truth. This stance of non-foundationalism emerged from my experiences. Life and learning are not simply developmental (growing into maturity, advanced learning stages or higher consciousness), but spatial and temporal. They are spatial in the sense that the discourses informing any context, and the subjectivities shaped by them, construct a geography of human relationships. I realized that to practise as a reconstructionist teacher was necessarily to avoid generalized theories of development or universalized understandings/truths. Such theories close down the possibilities inherent in any social space. In fact they are contrary to emancipatory practice, as they perpetrate the very thing that we are criticizing. I consider that the more people have access to many knowledge(s), the more the spaces open for a plurality of knowing (and therefore tolerance) in relationships.

As well as being spatial, life and learning are historically produced; hence my proposition of a narrative epistemology. I demonstrated with the use of a narrative form that there were other histories and other interpretations always present. Knowledge is multi-storied, never complete and always contingent. Opening the airwaves for multiple histories provides opportunities for the re-authoring of people's histories and therefore of students' learning and agency.

My thesis was a momentary, contingent and playful encounter with (my) theoretical passions of the present. I dreamed up and deconstructed a field of action in which the ironic tensions that are a part of any encounter between the might of the policy and governance of institutionalized education and the dynamism of an emancipatory project can play. The importance of an attitude of ironic tension was an outcome of the thesis. It emerged because radical forms of education are still positioned within the mainstream educational discourse, but the relationship between student and teacher is often more open in radical experiential education, and thus simultaneously works to defuse the discourse's objectifying tendencies. Categories such as student and teacher can become blurred and the possibility for agency more likely. Significantly, it is not only the student who changes. Constructing a piece of research that blurred the boundaries between life, research, teaching and learning also served to blur my personal edges. More specifically, negotiating the rules and regulations of dominant discourses and their social practices (like the rules of thesis writing) positioned me differently in relationship to them. Looking back on the creation of this thesis, I realize I recreated myself. I feel myself, in T. S. Eliot's (1963) words from the *Four Quartets*, 'returning to the beginning and knowing the place for the first time'. I have developed greater confidence, including a new-found uncertainty and set of paradoxes, in my work as a reconstructionist teacher. May the dance continue.

[1] A phrase used in *Re-authoring Lives* (White, 1990).

[2] Michel Foucault's oeuvre is extensive. I mainly drew on his work from *Discipline and Punish* (Foucault, 1977) onwards. Foucault's work is daunting to the new reader. There are many good starting texts written by others, for example, *Michel Foucault: Beyond Structuralism and Hermeneutics* (Dreyfus and Rabinow, 1983); *The Foucault Reader* (Rabinow, 1984); *Disciplining Foucault, Feminism, Power and the Body* (Sawicki, 1991).

[3] Process Oriented Psychology, an organization at the time centred in Switzerland (now USA) that was connecting the personal to the political through cross-cultural workshops/training in working with conflict/difference, held in a different country each year (Russia, Poland, India, Australia, South Africa). It is the brainchild of Arnold Mindell, author of, amongst other books, *Leader as a Martial Artist* (1992) and *Sitting in The Fire* (1995).

[4] This subject was called 'Learning Processes' and was in an undergraduate degree in the then School of Social Ecology, University of Western Sydney.

[5] Third-year students at the time embarked on a third-year project based on action research methodologies.

[6] Bourdieu's (1990) term.

[7] As it is in Aboriginal culture, I am using this phrase to refer to the manifest and non-manifest.

[8] I chose this title to capture the ironic tension that runs through this chapter, especially the first section. I later found it in *Changing Teachers, Changing Times* (Hargreaves, 1994).

[9] *Local Knowledge* (Geertz, 1983) is a collection of essays which strongly influenced this.

References

Bourdieu, P. (1990) *The Logic of Practice*. Cambridge: Polity Press.

Browning Cole, S. and Coultrap-McQuin, J. (1992) *Explorations in Feminist Ethics*. Indiana: Indiana University Press.

Byrne-Armstrong, H. (1999) Dead certainties and local knowledge: Poststructuralism, conflict and narrative practices in radical/ experiential education. PhD thesis, University of Western Sydney, NSW, Australia.

Dreyfus, H. and Rabinow, P. (eds) (1983) *Michel Foucault: Beyond Structuralism and Hermeneutics*, 2nd edn. Chicago: University of Chicago Press.

Eliot, T. S. (1963) *Collected Poems 1909–1962*. London: Faber & Faber.

Foucault, M. (1977) *Discipline and Punish: The Birth of a Prison*. London: Peregrine Books.

Foucault, M. (1983) Afterword: the subject and power. In *Michel Foucault: Beyond Structuralism and Hermeneutics*, 2nd edn (H. Dreyfus and P. Rabinow, eds), pp. 208–226. Chicago: University of Chicago Press.

Foucault, M. (1986) *The Care of the Self: The History of Sexuality*, Vol. 3. New York: Penguin Press.

Gebbie, T. (1994) On the subject of Postmodernism Feminism (unpublished).

Geertz, C. (1983) *Local Knowledge: Further Essays in Interpretive Anthropology*. New York: Fontana Press.

Gore, J. (1993) *The Struggle for Pedagogies: Critical and Feminist Discourses as Regimes of Truth*. London: Routledge.

Hargreaves, A. (1994) *Changing Teachers, Changing Times*. London: Cassell.

Horsfall, D. (1997) The subalterns speak: community health. PhD thesis, University of Western Sydney, NSW, Australia.

Irigaray, L. (1980) When our two lips speak together. *Signs*, **6**(1), 69–79.

Kreiger, S. (1991) *Social Science and the Self: Personal Essays on an Art Form*. New Jersey: Rutgers University Press.

Mindell, A. (1992) *Leader as a Martial Artist*. New York: Harper Collins.

Mindell, A. (1995) *Sitting in the Fire*. Portland: Lao Tse Press.

Nicholson, L. (1990) *Feminism Postmodernism*. New York: Routledge.

Polkinghorne, D. (1983) *Methodology for the Human Sciences*. New York: SUNY Press.

Polkinghorne, D. (1988) *Narrative Knowing and the Human Sciences*. New York: SUNY Press.

Rabinow, P. (1984) *The Foucault Reader*. New York: Pantheon.

Reinharz, S. (1992) *Feminist Methods in Social Research*. Oxford: Oxford University Press.

Salner, M. (1986) Adult cognitive and epistemological development in systems education. *Systems Research*, **3**(4), 223–232.

Sass, L. (1990) Humanism and hermeneutics. In *Hermeneutics and Psychological Theory: Interpretative Perspectives on Personality, Psychotherapy and Psychopathology* (S. Messer, L. Sass and R. Woolfolk, eds), pp. 222–271. New Jersey: Rutgers University Press.

Sawicki, J. (1991) *Disciplining Foucault, Feminism, Power and the Body*. New York: Routledge.

Stanley, L. (ed.) (1990) *Feminist Praxis: Research and Epistemology*. London: Routledge.

White, M. (1990) *Re-authoring Lives*. Adelaide: Dulwich Hill Press.

Section Three

The full Monty

6

Black holes in the writing process: narratives of speech and silence

Debbie Horsfall[1]

> *One must listen to her differently in order to hear an 'other meaning' which is constantly in the process of weaving itself, at the same time ceaselessly embracing words yet casting them off to avoid becoming fixed, immobilised. For when she 'says' something, it is already no longer identical to what she means. (Irigaray, in Weedon, 1987, p. 64)*

Sitting here in the study, with time to write, with having to write, streams of words are sucked into the black hole in my head; fierce words with all the power and energy of far off suns.

How come I decided to write this chapter? I never experience black holes in writing as I'm not that passionate!

I've got nothing worth saying.

I don't want to write about stuckness, how useful is that? I want to write about ways out of the stuckness, approaches that could be helpful.

I have absolutely no idea what a black hole is anyway, and even if I did what has it got to do with researching and writing? (Is it a black hole when the tools you need, or believe you need for writing just don't work? Is it irony that now I have the time to write this chapter, about stuckness in writing, I am in a house with no electricity and no computer? I don't write on paper, I write straight into the computer. So now what? Am I stuck, beaten by my own reliance on technology? Or is it that having panicked, then chilled out, I have not written but instead read, thought, talked about the writing, having been forced to resist my natural urge to sit down and physically write words on the page.)

This metaphor, of the black hole, is really problematic for me. Once again we are using a metaphor where 'black' is associated with something undesirable. In fact the adjective 'black' is what makes the 'hole' undesirable. Furthermore, coming from science, it seems that this is both a masculinist and racist metaphor – am I over-reacting?

Here we go again, into the 'process stuff' nothing substantial, no real content. How can I possibly write about process, when everybody's is so diverse? If I write about my own it will seem narcissistic, irrelevant and boring.

This subject has probably been 'done to death' by someone far cleverer, really famous and who writes passionately and beautifully.

Converging, connecting and coalescing, feeding each other, imploding into a mass of energy so dense that nothing can ever hope to break out.

This is miserable, hopeless, tortuous, I hate writing! I'm going down to the river to sulk. Mum's down there, perhaps I'll have a moan to her.
Perhaps she has felt like this too, maybe, I wonder ...

Slowly, almost imperceptibly, thoughts begin to weave themselves together. Turning around and around they gather energy and speed ...

It's really important to foreground writing about research, the 'writing up'. Writing is rarely, if ever, discussed as part of the labour process of researchers. Yet 'writing up' is a task we all have to do; whether as a report, a thesis, or an article, it is an integral part of the researching process. (Is this part of still seeing language as a neutral tool of re-presentation rather than as something we both create and are created by?) The writing is something we are just expected to be able to do, assumed to be able to do. Associated with this assumption is lack of clarity about what is expected, what exactly the rules are, how we can bend them if we want to. How insidious. How terrifying for those who are not keepers at the gate. No wonder we are often found with no words to write, with nothing worth saying

then break through the dense, seething mass ...

Part of writing is allowing ourselves to value the black hole, the 'sucking in' of our selves, our thoughts, our readings. This 'sucking in' could be supported if we who are writing 'academic' papers, theses, research reports could see our writing as a creative process. We could then work on valuing and privileging this creativity, this writing. In this valuing and privileging we would resist our histories and the scripts we play in/with our bodies – the ones that tell you to 'sit down' and 'start writing', that without words on a page you have 'not done any work' – and begin to value 'lying around writing', 'going for a walk writing', 'talking it over with friends/your mum writing', 'just hanging out writing'.[2]

About writing

> *Writing is my passion. Words are the way to know ecstasy. Without them life is barren. The poet insists language is a body of suffering, and when you take up language you take up suffering too. (hooks, 1997, p. 208)*

This chapter is not necessarily about untangling ideas and dropping them neatly into the lap of the reader. Hopefully, it is about exploring thoughts, passions and influences in relation to the process of writing research, in addition to giving voice to the stuckness that I, and many of the people I know, experience as I/they write. It also includes the imaginal as I ask, how could it be different? As I write/you read, I ask you to listen to me differently, while I strive for clarity and authenticity. I am not always able to say what I mean, and even when I do I know that I will not always remain fixed to my position of the moment. At the same time, I am aware that 'in an era of rampant reflexivity, just getting on with it may be the most radical action one can make' (Lather, 1991, p. 20).

Writing these words I am struggling/suffering with the question: How do I intervene in the 'production of knowledge at particular sites in ways that work out of the blood and spirit of our lives'? (Lather, 1991, p. 20). How do I speak of what influences my practice as a researcher/writer of research while at the same time avoiding the 'consumerism of ideas that can pass for the life of the mind in academic theory' (Lather, 1991, p. 20)? I am interested in *really useful knowledge*. By this I mean knowledge that helps me to understand and act in the world in ways that resist dominations, hierarchies, discriminations and oppressions. In moments of great hope and optimism (perhaps arrogance?) I also construct really useful knowledge as dreams, imaginings and ways of being which are transformative of the *status quo*.

There was a time when I found writing a chore, difficult, boring even. This was the time when I was worried about writing the right way, somehow proving I was 'academic' enough when I wrote. This meant sounding important, proving that I had read heaps of other people's words and saying nothing creative or original. I thought that when writing I had to tell the 'truth' and convince the reader that I was right, OK, not a fraud:

> *The clean sheet is so often faced with an anxiety invoked by a sense of the invisible authority of academic law. 'The paternal terror of Truth': will I speak the truth, in the name of the disciplinary Fathers? And what if I should stray? Have I got the correct thoughts together that will now be transcribed onto the page that awaits? (Game and Metcalfe, 1996, p. 93)*

Furthermore, as a woman I was/am not accustomed to claiming space for myself or believing that my voice is important, that I have something to say (Scutt, 1992, p. 3). What a great way to silence myself! Some of us seem to deal with this silencing by drying up, becoming blocked or disappearing into a jumble of words and waffle, not knowing how to both say enough and not say too much.

The bodily act of putting words on a page does frighten some of us. While we may talk freely with friends, colleagues or people in the street, this freedom of speech does not come so easily in the act of writing. In conversation there is chance to clarify, to change our minds, to retract, to illuminate. In writing these chances do not exist, there is a permanence to the words we speak. The words become frozen on the page and we are not so able to mediate the meanings others will make of what we say. In conversation there is an obvious relationship with the people with whom we are speaking. In writing this sense of relationship is not so apparent or obvious. Not having this more obvious relationship means that we have to be more careful as we write. We have to work out a way to write the conversation, with ourselves and our readers. At the same time we have to write according to different rules, or conventions, than when we speak. Writing asks that we sanitize out all the hesitations, the repetitions, the gestures used for emphasis and additional meaning, the half-finished sentences, our spoken idiosyncrasies.

> *Take a look at the words on this page. Forget, for a moment, what they are saying, and look at them as a pattern of letters and words arranged in a certain way. The arrangement is intensely logical. The words are ordered in a careful sequence: straight lines, one after the other, right down the page. There is an inherent rationality about the written word that is not present to the same extent in the ebb and flow of personal conversation ...*

When we chose the medium of print, we play by the rules of the medium. For a start, we will have to say everything we want in words alone. (Mackay, 1994, p. 267)

Playing by the rules of the medium becomes more complex as we consider the rules of the particular genre within which we are writing. A thesis is different to an essay is different to an article is different to a book chapter. Within each of these genres there are further rules or conventions. In the thesis or the essay these conventions are often discipline-bound. Writing in cultural studies will be different from writing in criminology or education. Students have always known that who they are writing for is important – knowing what the individual academic will accept/wants to hear, and then keeping upright as they teeter along the thin wavy line between telling the authority what it wants to hear and saying what they want to say. With writing an article for a journal, the conventions differ between journals. The editorial panel and peer reviewers will have different expectations of what type of style and content is 'acceptable', depending on the nature of the journal. The same can be said of book publishers. Then we move onto government departments. Often, especially in social research, we are hopeful that our 'findings' will have an impact on policy development and service provision. We have, then, to write up our research in a way that is acceptable to the bureaucrats. As writers of research it is our responsibility to find out what the particular rules and conventions are, to know to whom we are writing. When we know the rules and conventions, we can decide how closely we will follow them and how much we will push the boundaries.

The black hole: the politics of speech and silence

Often we are expected to write ourselves out of the story we are telling. We are expected to negate our bodies, our responses, our feelings, our dreams, our passions, and write in a cool, detached, disembodied manner. The report, the thesis, the article, the essay is assumed merely to represent and discuss the 'facts' about what we have 'found'. This assumption, often well grounded in reality, asks us to deny ourselves. This denial, especially for those who are struggling to find their voice, to believe that they have something to say that somebody will listen too, is death making. No wonder then, that the 'clean sheet' becomes the shroud that wraps us up in our own terror. We spiral into a black hole from which no breath, no words, no life can escape. To break out of this life-denying hole we need to understand the black hole, how we are held within it, while simultaneously growing the strength and courage to speak out, 'to break silence ... And given all the means by which silence is reinforced again and again, to break and re-break it' (Morgan, 1992, p. 18).

For some of us, breaking out of silence, taking up the suffering of which bell hooks speaks, requires a small amount of risk. We may risk sounding silly, not well enough informed, repetitive of what has already been said. We may be ridiculed, not heard, misunderstood. We may alienate those we are trying to impress. For others, saying the words out loud can mean expulsion from their country, imprisonment, torture or death. It can mean losing a job that earns money to put food on the table. It can mean that your children will be threatened and you live in constant fear. I say these words not to be overly dramatic. I know students and colleagues for whom these risks are not imagined and who live with fears I can barely imagine. For these people the acts of both silence and speech/writing require infinitely more exquisite struggle. Writing narratives of stuckness, in the way I do, comes from my position as a white, educated, middleclass woman who lives in a country where speaking out, from this position, is more of a psychological than material risk.

There is also a counter-narrative. Being sucked into the black hole, the 'cooking process', to mix my metaphors, is inseparable from the bodily act of writing. The ingredients need to be found, prepared and thrown into the pot to bubble away until ready to eat. We read, we think, we collect fragments of conversations. We mull over our field notes, our transcripts. We read reports and theses written by others for inspiration and perhaps clarity about how to structure the story. We talk with others about our researching. We try out some ideas with a few trusted friends to see if they somehow make sense. We may talk with the people with whom we researched, the people whose words in interviews, case studies and focus groups have given us much of our raw data. Only when we have reached saturation point, where we are discovering nothing new about what to say and how to say it, is the stew finally cooked and ready for the consumption of others. If at this point we are unable to spew the words onto the page, then we are truly stuck. Then we are not choosing silence: we are being silenced. We may be being silenced by an oppressive regime, where remaining silent is the only life-saving course of action, and/or our own histories and our position within society may be silencing us.

The distinction between choosing silence and being silent is an important one. Silence is often constructed as a passive, powerless action, coming from a place of oppression. While this may often be true, it is not always true. Choosing silence, not writing, at a point in time can be reconstructed as a position of power, 'power to define what is said and not said, heard and not heard ... power over the entire process of communication between us' (Morgan, 1992, pp. 189–190). Choosing silence is an expression, an act. To return to the metaphor of cooking, we would not knowingly serve under-cooked food to our guests. Similarly, many of us choose to not write under-cooked words out loud.

Many of us carry from childhood so-called words of wisdom that silence us: 'it's better to be thought a fool than to open your mouth and prove it'. We may struggle with a sense of not being good/creative/original/theoretical/practical/wonderful enough. Possibly this silencing began when we were told by someone in authority that what we said made no sense, that our words were not good enough, that we had not paid attention to our grammar and spelling. We became intimidated by what other people may think about our words, our voice.

As a small child I was always in the school choir. I loved to sing, and I loved the experience of making a loud noise with a group of people, of belting my voice out. When I was 10 or 11, my music teacher told me that I was 'tone deaf' and could no longer 'sing in tune'. Devastated, I became one of those people who mouthed the words of songs when expected to sing in public. I became embarrassed at the sound of my own voice. Recently I began to take singing lessons. In the first lesson my teacher asked me to follow her, with my voice, as she played notes on the piano. Terrified, hesitant, I did so. She turned to me, saying, 'there is nothing wrong with your ears, you can find the note and hold it, I can't imagine why anyone would tell you you can't sing!'. This puzzled me. We spoke more about what had happened. 'Seems to me', she said, 'that you are just afraid of the sound of your own voice, of making a loud noise and being heard!'. Shocked, I took these words away with me. It interested me that much of the work I do, in my researching and in my work with students, is concerned with people finding and having a voice, of not being silenced. I had some renewed understanding of the fear someone may experience when being asked to speak, to use their voice, orally or in writing.

It may be that we have a fear of both being heard and not being heard. Being heard is to do with being judged, being noticed, being misunderstood, being equated with our words, being held accountable for what we have said – being heard not singing in tune with those in authority.

> *These words have been brought forth with great care, risking more than a little and leaving me raw in the process.*
>
> *For fear.*
>
> *For being misunderstood. For fear of being misrepresented. For fear of never being answered.*
>
> *O beloved voice: have I just proven why you chose silence? (Morgan, 1992, p. 196)*

There are many tensions in writing, tensions that can be silencing. Many of these surface as we struggle with writing to the people who may read our work. 'The act of writing is addressing the silence of the unknown reader' (Morgan, 1992, p. 193). I am one of the readers for whom I write. In writing I clarify my thoughts, understand and know myself better. I also take a risk as I make myself visible to you and myself. In writing I make myself vulnerable. Imaginary readers 'in authority' who will judge this work, threaten nebulously. I write also for students and qualitative researchers who may read this work, to help them in writing their experience of researching. The tension, then, is in being true to myself and being accessible to others while at the same time being able to connect with, be understood and validated by those in authority. I experience this tension as a never-ending compromise. I have to be accepted, if I am to be heard, from both within and without. Thus I end up rarely saying what I really want to; the sharp, adversarial edges have by necessity been rubbed smooth. How do I write what I want to write, and still be heard? How do I hold these tensions and not disappear into a blank empty space of non-action?

Being silenced is an act of oppression. Some of us can resist this oppression and begin to speak out. I struggle against denying myself, silencing myself, shrouding myself. I will not pretend that meanings can be clearly presented, are transparent and clear. I will not act as if I have produced the knowledge and I am merely re-presenting it to you, dear reader. Knowledge has been/continues to be produced in the bodily act of writing of this chapter, in the many discussions and dialogues with friends and family along the way and in the relationship you will have with what is written. Writing this way and making this way visible is an act of resistance.

Writing is the passageway, the entrance, the exit, the dwelling place of the other in me – the other that I am and am not, that I don't know how to be, but that I feel passing, that makes me live. (Cixous, 1986, in Game and Metcalfe, 1996, p. 103)

As I reflect upon my researching, and the writing up of my PhD, I trace the development of my own voice. Understanding the black holes of writing, understanding how I had been both psychologically and socially constructed not to shout out loud, enabled me to begin the process of resistance and reconstruction. I began to work hard not to apologize for what I wanted to say, not to silence the fire in my voice. Much of what had kept me silent, in written form, was a belief that I was the same as everyone else, not much different and therefore I had nothing to say. I never knew I was 'other'. In fact I spent most of my time as a child trying to blend in, to become part of, the same as everyone else. This was not without challenges. My father was a Navy man, which meant that the family followed him around the country as he moved every 2–3 years. While part of me relished the opportunity constantly to reinvent myself, I was also conscious of always being the new kid on the block. Survival and the opportunity to develop friendships and be accepted meant that I had to learn quickly to be a chameleon and to adapt to the culture of the new place, to assimilate. I developed a range of strategies to blend in, not to be noticed, to become the same as. Looking back I am amazed at how successful I was at convincing myself that I was no different to anyone else. Believing that you are no different, that you blend in, can render you voiceless. What is there to say, why would anyone want to listen, surely we have heard it all before? Imagine the terror that this 'same as' person feels when asked to be original and creative.

It could be that the stuckness feels like slow strangulation as we struggle to write. Our voice is stifled, as too often we believe writing is merely a representation of the past, rather than our interpretation of the past/present. Believing this, we believe that there must be a right answer, a right way to write the 'truth'. This narrative oversimplifies the act of writing while at the same time rendering us silent. If we believe that writing is a representation, then, we may tell ourselves, it cannot be difficult to tell the story. At the same time we know that the world and our experience in and of it is far from simple. The other day my 14-year-old son was asked to write a review of the book he had finished reading. One of the first questions asked him briefly to explain the story of the book. He quickly became stuck, restless and angry. 'I can't do this,' he said, 'there are so many plots and subplots in this book, how can I explain them all?'. Part of his stuckness was realizing the complexity of what he understood and not knowing how to capture this complexity in writing. Another part of his stuckness was avoiding/resisting the hard work required to try and make some sense of the book as he briefly re-presented and reinterpreted it in his own words. I have a feeling that these two threads may have a lot to do with our own narratives of stuckness: knowing the tangled complexity of what we have 'found out', and knowing that it is going to be difficult to write this complexity. Part of this is due to the limitations of written language: we have only words, and words require linear construction. Our knowings, our understandings are often multifaceted, multidimensional and sometimes chaotic. And yet we are required to explain ourselves in one dimension; there is no room for the multitude of voices, thoughts and feelings that occur in the meaning-making in our bodies.

A sense of purpose

> *In 1991, the world learned of a recently discovered ancient language devised at least one thousand years earlier in a mountainous region of the Hunan Province in central China.*
>
> *It was a totally female language ...*
>
> *'Nushi' ('women's writing') used characters derived from standard Chinese to represent the syllables of the local dialect. Standard Chinese has no such phonetic base; it uses characters pictographically, to represent meaning only. Chinese linguists believe that the women developed the script because they were forbidden to learn standard writing ... for hundreds of years women used the script to record their hidden emotions and to communicate with each other surreptitiously ...*
>
> *One Nushi author wrote, 'Men leave home to brave life in the outside world. But we women are no less courageous. We can create a language they cannot understand'.*
>
> *These were the words of a woman who might as well have written, 'We shall not suffer in silence'. Because this female language was an underground code – an act of rebellion in conception, an utterance of rebellion in content. (Morgan, 1992, pp. 276–277)*

Perhaps we are silenced by not understanding why we are writing. Many of the research students I work with are social activists. They are working with issues such as sexual abuse, marginalization within the health system, supporting families from materially poor backgrounds, working with children deemed 'at risk'. Many of these students see the purpose of their work as taking action against oppressions and discriminations, being in the 'thick of it'. They construct writing as a non-action, as not changing the lived experiences of the people for whom and with whom they work. 'When one is writing, why isn't one "at the barricades"?; when one is at the barricades, why isn't one writing?' (Morgan, 1992, p. 16). Often people working as social activists take the position of advocate with/for oppressed people. Adding to, inserting one's voice into the 'body of knowledge' seems a far way off from the immediacy of the appalling conditions many people live with daily. I have some understanding of this position, having worked in the 'community sector' for many years, and I have certainly struggled with the 'indulgences' of writing.

I wonder, though, what is really going on here, when we accept the dualism of acting and writing. There seems to be an issue of reverse elitism. Intellectual work, the writing up of the research, is seen as irrelevant. The real work occurs at the barricades, in the streets and refuges. Writing only takes one away from the work of the revolution. How can we resist this construction? To see that when working at the barricades one is doing intellectual work, and when writing one is being a social activist? Both are acting in the world; it is the nature of the action, what one is doing with one's body that differs. Writing and being at the barricades can be political acts if one's purpose is to unsettle, question and destabilize the *status quo*. 'Politics in the most profound sense is not restricted to deals made in the halls of the powerful or demonstrations marched in the streets of the powerless' (Morgan, 1992, p. 15).

The writing/acting dualism, between intellectual work and street work, serves to silence social activists themselves. Another tyranny takes place, one that does serve the interests of the activists or the people for/with whom they advocate. Not writing about what we know, what we have found, what we experience, we run the risk of falling:

> *... prey to be written about, distorted, erased, simplified, analysed or compartmentalized by a new crop of 'objective' historians with their own hidden political agendas – whether conservative, Marxist, male supremacist, or simply boring. So it becomes even more crucial to tell our own story. (Morgan, 1992, p. 14)*

Writing becomes another act of resistance and reconstruction in the process of transforming the world in which we live. Writing our own stories of the work that we do means that we are resisting allowing an 'authority', whose interests may not coincide with our own, to write our stories for us.

Story-telling/narrative

> *Blending colours,*
> *Weaving fragments together,*
> *Making music,*
> *Choreographing a dance ... (McCutcheon, 1993)*

Writing is a creative activity. Some may argue that writing up researching is merely re-presentation of what happened, when, how and what we found out. I say that there is always an act of creation and creativity, we 'stitch things up as we write up the world' (Jaki Nidle-Taylor, personal communication). There is an art to writing, the artfulness of creative and careful conversations with words on the page.

> *While the facts of scientists and the fiction of novelists are created under significantly different disciplinary constraints, both try to simulate and tell truths about a world to which neither has unmediated access. (Game and Metcalfe, 1996, p. 63)*

When I was searching for a structure for my PhD thesis, a way to represent researching, I remembered a conversation with a friend and colleague, Hilary. She had recently completed her Masters Honours thesis, and was talking of her struggle to find her own voice. She worked through this struggle by thinking of her work as a story, and chose to 'just write the story, my story, as that is all it is – a story' (Hilary Armstrong, personal conversation; see also Byrne-Armstrong, 1990). Such profound simplicity can be inspiring and empowering. Talking of 'telling stories' as a way to write about our researching could seem to trivialize the work that we do. I would contest this. Telling a story, or using a narrative approach, is a way of organizing what we want/need to say. The story connects the events that took place. 'Stories connect events in time. In Forster's formulation their basic structure is "And then ... And then ... And then ... " (1962)' (Game and Metcalfe, 1996, p. 68). Isn't this what we are doing as we write up researching? We use our imagination and creativity to select and organize 'events', 'facts', 'findings'. These we weave together in a linear way to re-present our researching as a coherent process, bound in time, which some-how will make sense to our selves and our readers. In doing this we begin to order the often chaotic lived experience of researching. In writing our story of researching we translate and recreate our 'jumble of experience' (Game and Metcalfe, 1996, p. 76).

Using a narrative/story-telling approach to write my research allowed me to discover my voice and a way of writing the thesis. Writing in this way enabled me to know writing as a process of translation, re-presentation and creation. I immersed myself in the craft of weaving words together to tell the story of my researching. Somehow it's all about telling a story. We become the storytellers, telling a story that encourages conversations, thoughts and feelings, as well as presenting the 'facts' of our researching. Re-framing writing as story-telling also lets me see that what I am writing is only truth-in-the-moment, as I know that 'there is no absolute truth when it comes to how we remember the past' (hooks, 1997, p. xix, quoting Lorde).

Holding the idea of writing our research as a story gave me some organiz-ing questions, a structure:

- What sort of story is it?
- What is the story about?
- Are there any subplots, smaller stories captured in the bigger story?
- Who are the main characters, what role/s do they play, why are they important to the story and what does the reader need to know about them?
- What were the significant events/happenings? How do they fit?
- Where is the story set, what is the scenery, the props?
- What does the reader need to know in order to make some sense of the story?
- Does the story need to be told as it actually happened, to be true to the chronology of events, or is there some creative licence around this?
- Is it a story to invite the reader in, to engage them in some way?

The writing of this chapter is also telling a story. Writhing out of my own narratives of stuckness I have told you fragments of my story as I struggled to write about my own researching. Interwoven are the stories of people important to me: friends, family, colleagues and students. I have also woven in some threads of the larger story of the society and culture that shapes, strangles our voices. I have re-presented some 'facts', the lived experiences of the people I know, in addition to using my imagination and creativity to select content, form and purpose. As qualitative researchers, each one of us has a story to tell, and each story is something of importance.

As we write up our researching we need to be both humble and coura-geous, knowing that all we can do is capture a moment in time and say, 'this is my story, I've told it, and in your hands I leave it' (Warner, 1994, p. xxi).

This is the humility, knowing that our voice, when we find it, is one of many. Knowing that what we know is only a partial story of the world. Knowing that we must insert our own partial stories, so that we are not silenced, marginalized, trivialized or rewritten by another. As we hold this humility, we also develop our courage. It takes courage to speak up and out. Often writing our researching is 'work done at the limits of ourselves' (Foucault, 1984, p. 46) as we are constructing a resistance story, creating mobile and transitory points of resistance (Foucault, 1980) through our thinking and writing, knowing that resistance is difficult.

Writing, telling the story, is taking action. While writing includes commentary and re-presentation of our researching, it is more than this. We write the relationships and connections of our everyday stories of researching within the larger stories of our cultures and the societies in which we live. Writing is an act that enables us to define our worlds, our cultures and our experiences in our own words. Writing is an act against being silenced.

[1] With thanks to Ann Smith, Andy Horsfall and Jaki Nidle-Taylor, with whom I did the 'talking it over with friends/your mum writing'.
[2] Thanks to Susan Murphy for these ideas originally in relation to researching.

References

Byrne-Armstrong, H. (1990) Spinning the threads of Indira's net: reflexivity in action. MSc(Hons) thesis, University of Western Sydney, Hawkesbury, NSW, Australia.

Foucault, M. (1980) *Power/Knowledge; Selected Interviews and Other Writings 1972–1977 by Michel Foucault* (C. Gordon, ed.). London: Harvester Press.

Foucault, M. (1984) What is enlightenment? In *The Foucault Reader* (P. Rabinow, ed.), p. 10. New York: Pantheon.

Game, A. and Metcalfe, A. (1996) *Passionate Sociology*. London: Sage.

hooks, b. (1997) *Wounds of Passion: A Writing Life*. London: The Women's Press.

Lather, P. (1991) *Getting Smart: Feminist Research and Pedagogy with/in the Postmodern*. London: Routledge.

Mackay, H. (1994) *Why Don't People Listen?* Sydney: Pan Macmillan.

McCutcheon, M. (1993) Writing ecologically (unpublished paper).

Morgan, R. (1992) *The Word of a Woman*. London: Virago Press.

Scutt, J. A. (1992) *As a Woman Writing Women's Lives*. Melbourne: Artemis.

Warner, M. (1994) *From the Beast to the Blonde: On Fairy Tales and Their Tellers*. Sydney: Random House.

Weedon, C. (1987) *Feminist Practice and Poststructuralist Theory*. Oxford: Blackwell.

7

Fragile relationships[1]

Alma Fleet, Susan Holland, Barbara Leigh and Catherine Patterson

Scanning the sea

Researching education at doctoral level may seem to be a straightforward academic exercise, primarily of interest to those who choose to undertake that research because of the contribution to the career path of the researcher and to the knowledge base of the discipline. However, as with most aspects of human endeavour, when this activity is itself put under the research microscope, interesting, multi-layered realities emerge.

We, the authors of this chapter, are familiar with the rigours and rituals involved in this type of academic work, since each of us has at some time in the past decade successfully completed a doctoral programme. Our separate and collective experiences and those of other women, which we detail below, suggest that doctoral work can be best understood when viewed not as an isolated or singular pursuit of predetermined academic processes but as an integrated and richly layered set of lived research experiences. Our purpose here is to portray, accurately and compassionately, the nature of the doctoral research experience, and specifically a critical and very pivotal aspect of that experience: the relationship between researcher and supervisor.

For us and for others from whom we have collected data, this relationship is inherently fragile. All interpersonal relationships, whether of an intimate, loving kind in the personal domain or of a practical kind in the work domain, have the potential to be fragile because of the unique set of attributes and strength of character each person can bring to bear on the other. In addition, the supervisor relationship in the research domain has two features that make it unlikely that the relationship can ever be very robust. First, there is the unequal status of the researcher and the supervisor, which creates an asymmetrical power situation; and secondly, there is the length of time over which the relationship has to be sustained – even for full-time candidates, a minimum of three years.

We have structured this chapter using metaphors relating to the sea for, as with the movement of water, our lived research experiences have been characterized by the cycle of ebb and flow, the turbulence of competing forces and the exhilaration of being carried along, just for a short time, without the usual effort. At the beginning there is exploration (scanning the sea) as well as finding the courage to get started (taking the plunge). The selection of a supervisor and engagement in the research process follows (helping, hindering and swimming alone). At last there is some exhilaration (riding the waves) before the final outcome from the examination process (diving deep and surfacing). Afterwards life goes on, but not as before (charting new waters).

In recent years the experience of women in the academy has become an area of legitimate research interest because, having been ignored for so long, it can now be taken as an interesting problematic to be explored. However, the experience of graduate women as learners has not as yet been investigated in any great detail (Hayes and Flannery, 1997). Given that education as a discipline has been particularly welcoming to women entering its professional levels as teachers but not necessarily supportive of them in its scholarly halls, we anticipated that there would be value, at least for those who follow us, in describing fully the learning and development processes, positive and negative, objective and subjective, rational and emotional, which contribute to the doctoral experience in this discipline from the perspective of women.

This study began many years ago with friendly conversations among a group of women involved in doctoral programmes who were sharing a small, sparsely furnished tower room with other graduate students in a Faculty of Education. As the women had full and complex lives apart from their research, they talked to keep their sense of humour and preserve their sanity as they struggled to balance priorities and meet deadlines. Since several of these students were already working full-time in professional positions, the members of the group were rarely all in the room at the same time. At one time, the conversation centred on the most effective way to get photographs into a thesis that was due immediately. At another, there was book slamming and anger about a fruitless discussion with a supervisor. There were shared excitements about developments in an ethnographic project overseas, and then about a set of transcripts coded for discourse analysis. As the group continued their diverse studies with solid determination, they decided that their voices needed to be heard. They became conscious that they and other women doctoral students were operating in a world that did not acknowledge them as persons with multiple roles and responsibilities; nor were their methods of study or research questions necessarily being given due attention. So they laughed about being 'women at the top', who were simply at the top of a flight of stairs. Now many of them are, in fact, at the top of their professions. That transition and the steps up that tower are the foundation of this study.

In the intervening time, the field of women's studies has matured and now spans most disciplines. As a result there is a wide range of descriptions of feminism. We prefer Spendiff's (1992, p. 109) concept of feminism as 'the struggle of women to decide for ourselves what we want to be'. In this study, in paraphrasing Spendiff, our focus is on placing *women and the experience of women* centrally on the doctoral education agenda.

We draw on the experience in Australia of fifteen women, including ourselves, who were working on their doctoral studies in education in the 1980s. Most of us completed our theses in the early 1990s, although one chose to withdraw from the field and her study altogether. In reporting on our experiences, this study draws on relevant literature, two sets of questionnaires, a number of interviews, focus group discussions, journal entries and memories. It is not a tidy study, but neither were our experiences discreet or systematic. Our study both describes the research experience and analyses these experiences, highlighting emerging themes for the interest of other researchers and for women who may be considering doctoral study.

The Australian nature of the experience adds an important dimension. In contrast with many of the experiences reported from North America, the women in this study did not move 'naturally' into doctoral study as a logical follow-on (*cf.* Neumann, 1997) from previous university study. Rather, research often emerged after a break of some years of employment and/or time spent fulfilling family responsibilities. As a result the women initially found themselves working in isolation, not as members of a cohort, a formal study group, or even an informal network.

All of us began our studies at different times and for unique reasons. There was no common graduation or joyful celebration. Each of us is a survivor; while some were strategic others merely persisted. The most common experience of the doctoral journey was one of a constant struggle, requiring courage to overcome false fears as well as determination to succeed despite many frustrations. It is important to note that it has been several years since the writers completed their theses. This time has been necessary to achieve distance from the emotional power of the experience, to establish new or evolving careers, and to undertake the reflection necessary in the debriefing of self as case study.

The stories we explore in this chapter move between data and anecdote, reference and reminiscence. The value of personal narrative as data has been recognized in a range of areas (LePage and Flowers, 1995; Elbaz-Luwisch, 1997), as has the power of 'a collective of co-researchers' (Crawford *et al.*, 1990, p. 336). For us the value of this study lies in the resonance of the interrelated voices that nonetheless tell their own story, rather than in the logical report of an implied linear process. Our intent is to put the lived experiences into a shared framework and an accessible research context. Above all, we try to avoid oversimplification, that academic tendency to generalize which can misrepresent the complexity of the events, behaviours, motivations and feelings being investigated.

At this stage in our reflective and collaborative work the following themes have emerged: the fragile nature of the supervisor/student relationship, the value of memory within our methodological approach, the critical role of emotions in the learning process, and the legitimate and affirming power of the personal journey irrespective of the professional outcome. Our stories suggest that the doctoral journey can be conceptualized as consisting of two complementary dimensions: an objective, intellectual orientation which shapes the methodology and the research questions, and a less well defined but important subjective, emotional current which carries the tension as well as the energy and enthusiasm to sustain the journey. The personal journey moves along as a more or less positive or negative experience in fluid episodic waves. In our view, the gender and personality factors embedded in the supervisory relationship have powerful roles in shaping the progress of the journey.

Taking the plunge

Each story in this chapter is unique. There is no blueprint for success, or list of suggestions to be followed. These stories emerge from moments of critical reflection, sometimes bitter, and yet always creative and compassionate. They are personal reflections on key aspects of the research process, with a focus on relationships with supervisors and the experience of the examination process within the context of the doctoral journey. For some of the group of women it was a positive, enriching experience; for others it was a constant source of tension and conflict in which regaining power and control became a necessary precursor to successful completion.

Overall, our different memories remind us that the doctoral journey for women was as much an emotional and as a professional experience:

I enjoyed the intellectual stimulation . . .

I felt the work needed to be done and it was very challenging . . .

Despite all – I think the data is exciting and the project is worthwhile

I have a sense of exhilaration as I work on it . . .

It's like a millstone around my neck, but at the same time it's very interesting

I have something to say and I want to say it to the best of my ability

So, why did this group of women begin doctoral study? In their words:

I was tired of missing jobs . . .

There was also my personal pride because so many idiots (males) had PhDs

Job/employment prospects plus boredom at work . . .

I wanted the stimulation and a senior lectureship . . .

My husband was undertaking research and I wished to undertake postgraduate study concurrently

I have implemented a programme and wanted to know what it was that made parents and children see it so positively

I wanted to prove I had the intellectual capacity . . .

Some were strategic: they wanted a promotion. Others who had been passed over in job interviews wanted the requisite qualification, a doctorate. On the other hand, perhaps because of the empowering nature of education *per se*, many had broader purposes based on the intrinsic value they placed on the potential of their chosen research to increase the knowledge base, expand the professional field or enrich people's lives. On reflection, during interviews and focus group processes many of us perceived an integral link between the power of knowledge which might come from our research, and the need for the research to be done so that the world might be a better, fairer, more just place. Even in the initial motivation the personal dimension was evident. In fact, our collective memory suggests that it was this personal, subjective self that generated the self-confidence, the pride in achievement and the determination to keep producing. For one of us, though, the frustration with an inept and unsympathetic supervisor was so intense that opting out was ultimately seen as the saner course of action.

The student/supervisor relationship characterizes the dynamic nature of the doctoral process. These relationships were not static. While as graduate researchers we began optimistically, and looked forward to the guidance, support and intellectual challenge we expected from our respective supervisors, few of the supervisory relationships actually remained positive throughout the period of candidature. Rather, most of us experienced difficulties in the supervisory relationship, particularly as we moved from the position of novice to that of experienced researcher.

The following section includes the recall of critical moments as the voices of the women in our group tell how the intimate and therefore very personal nature of the supervisory process impacted on them emotionally as well as in their professional lives as doctoral students. The journey begins with the selection of a supervisor and then moves on to explore some of the complexities of the developing supervisory relationship. Finally, the journey ends with accounts of the examination experience and a look into possible futures.

Helping, hindering and swimming alone

Choosing a supervisor was sometimes a deliberate and strategic process, while in other cases the pairing with a supervisor seemed almost accidental. Early positive impressions were often revised as the relationships developed. For example, one woman stated:

> *I first met my supervisor during my Masters course. He was one of my lecturers. I was very interested in the research work that he was doing and I thought this is the person that I need to have as my supervisor. I did not realize then that you need to check interpersonal qualities as well as management qualities in choosing a supervisor. I just went for someone I respected intellectually who was working in an area that ignited my interest. I didn't think about the other issues, nor did I know then that he had not previously supervised doctoral students.*

The beginning of the supervisory relationship had elements of mentoring in a few cases and systematic guidance in others. Only one woman commented on a social component in the doctoral experience:

> *... he was wonderfully hospitable, he and his wife. He was more of a colleague, but at the same time, I respected him, I respected his intellect and I respected the fact that anyone with a PhD thesis was meant to act like him. He taught in a way that we would expect. That's how colleagues and researchers work together. And that's how you worked with him. And he'd play tennis with you. I know his kids ... I've been to his house. That kind of interaction is welcome.*

At times, however, many of the women felt they were swimming alone towards their goal. To maintain the momentum of their studies, several women commented that they had the responsibility of initiating meetings with their supervisor. One woman noted:

My supervisor didn't initiate anything. Initially there were a few meetings scheduled when I would go and make excuses. Then, he would let it drift and I would also let it drift. I could have died and gone to heaven, and neither the supervisor nor the university would have noticed.

In contrast, another woman commented that if her supervisor had not heard from her for some time, he would call to arrange a meeting. She would then feel obliged to schedule the meeting weeks in advance to give herself time to make progress on her thesis, as he always expected written evidence of work.

Many of the group experienced positive elements within the supervisory relationship, although only three felt that their overall experiences of supervision were satisfactory. Examples of statements from these three include:

I expected him to provide strategic advice regarding the structure of the thesis, methodology and so on. He also suggested an important conceptual framework to help situate the research (or part of it) that I would not have thought of and this becoming central to the thesis and my future academic work.

It was fine – it was just a professional relationship ...

This unrelieved patience with my intellectual struggle was certainly foreign to what I had ever encountered before in my relationship with authority figures at various workplaces. This caring, non-judgmental approach sustained me.

The more common experiences of supervision, however, are illustrated by the following:

I was expecting a collegial relationship. This wasn't met. I was treated as an inferior at times, keeping me waiting for my appointment while he finished work on the computer.

I expected more warmth, more knowledge, more praise. Part of my learning was learning to accept her as she is and the fact that we would never be friends.

Another example illustrates changes in the relationships over time:

Initially, I was very happy with the supervisory relationship. But towards the end, following his return from sabbatical, it was very unsatisfactory. I was unsure as to whether he was my supervisor or whether I had been transferred permanently to the temporary supervisor. I was caught between two protagonists. I felt let down by him, particularly with his lack of empathy re. the anxiety I was experiencing about whose advice I should follow.

Or there were evidences of disappointment which were almost tangible:

I explained to him that I had felt directionless during my Masters thesis (with a rather distant female supervisor) and was looking for more interaction. I thought he understood; in any case he didn't challenge that notion. The friendly, intellectually stimulating relationship I had in mind never eventuated. Although he arranged study space, meeting times and some funding (the full value of which I didn't appreciate until recently), these were systemic assistance, rather than collegial conceptualizing. I may have been visualizing something that wasn't possible.

The sense of disquiet that emerges from these voices was common throughout the interviews. At its most extreme, the lack of control and a feeling of powerlessness in one dysfunctional relationship ultimately generated so much anger that it became a catalyst for dramatically changing the situation and resolving some of the underlying conflicts:

> And the first thing I had to do was to change the way I related to my supervisor, I had to get some controls in place and I had to stop behaving like a victim. I had to stop having this submissive attitude, 'I don't understand until you tell me', 'until you give me a tick, it is not going to be any good', and 'you are never going to give me tick so it is never going to be any good', 'so I'll just keep going backwards, and in the meantime I'll keep feeling guilty'. So I had to take charge and put in some controls.

In other cases, the anger was never dealt with, nor the conflict resolved.

Personality factors and individual differences shaped many aspects of supervisory relationships. While gender issues were implied, none of the respondents initially 'praised' or 'blamed' gender factors for any aspect of their academic journey. With further prompting, however, more than half of the women commented on gender issues in the supervisory relationship. Only two said that they preferred to have a female supervisor. One of them wrote:

> I am very pleased to have a female supervisor. That may be my own personal predilection. I enjoy working with men, but I would want to have a female supervisor; now that's a little paradox you have to live with.

Another woman explained that she had had three male and two female supervisors. She felt that the men 'didn't really know how to handle a female academic at that level doing a PhD'. Nevertheless, she also stated that of the two women, one was 'too soft' and the other was 'too tough', so for her, too, gender factors were paradoxical.

One woman who identified gender as a relevant factor noted that she preferred to work with a male supervisor because 'the issue of experience, power and influence was important'. In contrast, one of the group said that gender did not play a factor in the supervisory relationship, and that 'I was more impressed by his status and promotion within the faculty'.

The issue of gender itself is not constant, but is embedded in the unique characteristics of each relationship, as highlighted by the following reflective comments:

> I think he was more comfortable with the male students around at the time, but it may have been a personality clash, or a stylistic difference, rather than purely gender.

> My first supervisor (female) and I used to talk a great deal about things other than my doctorate ... the second supervisor (male) was very much the master of the situation.

> But there was a feeling early, that this [PhD land] was boys' country.

> Following the breakdown of our supervisory relationship, I think he put it down to a 'neurotic woman' type explanation.

Another perspective came from one woman who was comfortable with the notion of a male supervisor because she valued people for who they were, rather than having stereotypical expectations of a relationship. In retrospect, however, she felt that the communication breakdown that occurred would have been far less likely if the supervisor had been less overpowering and more collegial, and that perhaps she would have been more comfortable with a female supervisor. In another situation, one woman reported that the gender of her supervisor affected her choice of thesis topic. She began her doctoral studies with a female supervisor who was very supportive of her work on a feminist perspective on change processes. When she transferred to another university because of a change in her partner's employment, she found herself working with a male supervisor who, although supportive, was not comfortable with such a feminist orientation and subsequently her study took a different direction. The issue of gender may have been more problematic than some of the women were willing to acknowledge.

So what sustained these women to keep battling the currents? The need for recognition, the thrill of the ride, or the compelling force of pragmatic reason to finish what was started? The answers are complex, multi-layered and intensely personal. The voices of the women who shared their experiences with us suggest there were internal as well as external drivers that sustained the lonely journeys, which in several cases wound over many more years than initially expected. These were journeys that tested relationships, provoked strong emotions and yet generated a deep sense of satisfaction for all but one of the women interviewed.

Riding the waves

The analogy of riding the waves evokes a feeling of euphoria. The crest that one rides at such a moment is so high that often before that moment of exhilaration, one flounders in the water and wonders whether attaining the crest will ever be possible. Riding the waves depicts the formal end to a long process. The other part of the analogy is that one is not yet to shore, hasn't completely arrived. There is the very real possibility of falling back into the ocean, even at this late stage. The euphoria is conditional, and there are others who will determine the final outcome. The final element to riding the waves is that in the case of women researchers in education, it is highly probable that their supervisors and the majority of their examiners will be male. Proving that one is 'equal to the task' often has a sexual component, usually at a quite deep unspoken level. When this group of female researchers did our PhDs, access to women supervisors was limited, and the relationship (usually with a male supervisor) was one that was, of necessity, on a one-to-one basis. Our awareness that the 'great man' image could be projected onto a supervisor or an examiner was an issue we discussed. Similarly, the disgust that was felt with male academics whose only interest was in career advancement was also raised. Riding the crest is a physical act that is saying, 'I made it!'. It is an analogy for what is not just a cerebral journey, but is in fact a process that takes place on many different levels.

In the examination process in Australia, three examiners are chosen, of whom usually one is internal and one is external to the institution, whilst the third may be either. Although the supervisor has the formal responsibility to choose the examiners, liaison with the student indicates the desire for this process to be as smooth and as intellectually profitable as possible. The following comments highlight the different emphases given to the process. In some cases the emphasis was strategic: 'Let's choose someone who will pass the thing!'. In others the emphasis was on showing one's colours: 'Let's choose the most famous people we can in this field!'. Of course this was not an either/or choice, but the different emphases did indicate feelings of the PhD student (and her supervisor) about her work. The following exemplifies the strategic approach:

> *I was very strategic in arranging examiners. Unlike the rest of my PhD experience, I was very much in charge of this process. I had a set of criteria for choosing the examiners and my supervisor supported me. The list was atypical in that I didn't want anyone outside Australia, I wanted at least one woman, and I wanted someone who was sympathetic to the methodological base I had used.*

Another woman was more concerned that her work be put on an international table of repute and be judged a success. Unfortunately in this instance her aim backfired. Nonetheless, her primary concern was with proving herself in the highest possible academic arena:

> *There was a world expert in my area whom I did not contact personally all the time I was doing my thesis, and I badly wanted him as an examiner. I nominated him, of course, but just at that time he decided to go mountain climbing. In retrospect, it would have been more valuable to consult him earlier and receive input throughout the study. But I wanted to have a world expert as my examiner.*

For someone else, however, the process of choosing examiners was frustrating, as all her suggestions were ignored. 'Riding the waves' was not going to come easily:

> *I felt the whole thing was testing from beginning to end. I never really got over the fact that I was being made to jump through every hoop in the system.*

Another woman, who also found the process of choosing examiners to be a manifestation of an underlying difficult relationship with her supervisor, experienced a similar reaction:

> *At this stage, I suspected that my major supervisor was not confident about the quality of my work. I certainly felt he had given inadequate guidance. No doubt each of us thought that the other had not made an appropriate contribution to ensuring a top quality product ... In my case, thinking back to my discussions with my supervisor on examiners, they seem, like most of the memories of supervisory exchanges, to be rather uncomfortable, if not actually tense.*

The euphoria of a process completed is felt at different stages, and sometimes not at all. For one of the group, it was graduation day that was important. The importance of significant others (in this case the parents) and the notion of 'making it' coalesced:

> *But my graduation day – ah, that was one of the best days of my life. It was close to Easter and my mother and father came over from New Zealand for a holiday and they were able to attend the ceremony. They had never been to one of my graduations and none of my three brothers had completed a university degree, so this was a new experience for them. I really felt as though I had made it.*

Unlike the supervisory process of the PhD, in which so many of the meetings are just between two people in an office, the examination process is a very public happening. Our research has exposed the fragility of the earlier relationship. However, by the time one is riding the wave, the relationship between supervisor and student often changes. As one respondent stated, 'I felt more of a peer when we chose the examiners'. As noted above, another woman remembered being in 'control mode'.

As those of us who have moved into academia are only too well aware, the examination process turns a strong light not just upon the student but also upon the supervisor. Students are often unaware of the sometime fragile egos of their supervisors. Such understanding comes with maturity.

The reaction of the student to the examination reports is one that we have tried to assess. In recalling this stage of the doctoral journey, many of us became aware of subjective as well as cognitive responses. In one instance, response to negative feedback in a report was given undue weight, even though the thesis did not require rewriting. Respondents often expressed the feeling of insecurity, not as a total emotional reaction but as one that surfaced from time to time and influenced perceptions of self. The fact that this carried right through to the examination process is indicative of how some students are afraid to claim their success without very strong and constant reinforcement. We wondered whether women are more susceptible in this area than men:

> *My experience in receiving my examiners' reports was one in which I believed only the critical comments (that came from an American male whom I knew) and tended to disregard the laudatory comments (that came from an interstate female whom I also knew) . . . Only now [six years later] am I feeling real merit in the work that I undertook. At the time, the task of completing a PhD was not about advancing in my career, but about proving something to myself. Once the process was over, I did not lay claim to the content as an academic might, but mentally pushed it aside as a task that was now done.*

In another instance, a woman remembers with disappointment the brevity of the reports. They were each positive, but were only two to three paragraphs in length. Despite the fact that they noted a 'pioneering approach' and a 'philosophical understanding', it was their brevity that was remembered.

The examination process is one that usually leads to 'riding the waves', but does not necessarily do so. One of our respondents decided that the PhD process was not for her, and left. For many, the time between submission and the receiving of the examiners' reports was one of great self-doubt. When the reports finally came in, one woman remembered the time as a 'home straight' where minor details dominated. 'I got the white-out and thought to myself, so it all comes down to this.' For her, the feeling of riding the waves came years later. Just as the waves merge into the ocean, so too does the fragility of relationship between supervisor and student in the writing phase merge into the examination stage. The waves are stronger and more powerful close to the shore, and riding on their crests with a completed PhD can send reverberations into all significant relationships. Fragility may thus become a little stronger, with ripples occurring years later.

Diving deep and surfacing

To divorce the personal value of the PhD from other inner journeys is somehow to sterilize it, sanitize it and remove it to the realm of the cognitive and the academic. We wish to challenge those divides. It is in the recognition that learning (including the PhD) involves the emotions (Arnold, 1994) that we can better understand (or name) processes and layers of the journey, and possibly better prepare the way for those that follow. A brief look at the wider ocean may make clearer the seascape in which the journeys are based.

As with other structured experiences, there are as many stories as there are people who have lived through the experience. The PhD is one of our society's revered institutions, yet the rules and regulations of what is permissible and what is beyond the bounds have been set up relatively recently. The first PhD in Australia was awarded at the University of Melbourne in April 1948. Surprising as it may seem, this first PhD was awarded to a woman, Erica Wolff, for her biographical and literary summary of the life and work of the French Australian writer Paul Wenz (Evans, 1998).

The PhD educational process adopted by Australian universities was taken from the English model of Oxford and Cambridge. It is one that relies on a great deal of self-motivation and inner generation of the topic. The supervisor is placed in the position of mentor and guide, which is conducive to a great deal of cooperation and sharing of interest if the supervisor is mature and has the time and the requisite shared interest in the topic.

This somewhat exclusive relationship between supervisor and student is different from the American model, where the student is required to undertake course work for the PhD and the dissertation is presented to a committee and is not the full requirement for the degree. The glimpses of the relationships we have included here suggest that in these Australian experiences the concept of supervisor as mentor was not a universal model.

Today there are even more reasons why the supervisor/mentor model is 'cracking at the seams'. The first has to do with the dramatic increase in PhD students within Australian universities in all faculties, including education, over the last two decades. The push-up effect of educational expansion (Craig and Spear, 1982) has led to the currency of the PhD being in great demand. At the same time as this increase has been occurring, there has been a corresponding shrinking of academic resources to handle the increase. Non-tenured staff have been terminated in an attempt to meet the demands of governments which have allocated less money to the university sector in what they feel are national priorities (or, if one is cynical, vote-buying priorities). Meanwhile, the remaining staff members take on increasing loads of undergraduate teaching, research and administration. Therefore, the environment in which a student enters a doctoral programme at the turn of the century is one in which a supervisor may be extremely stretched for time and the student can expect to be juggling an income-generating activity while coping with personal crises at various points of the research.

The second reason that the supervisor/mentor model is cracking at the seams has to do with the knowledge/information explosion which makes it difficult to keep abreast of a small field, let alone keep up to date in one's reading of a range of publications appearing around the world in cognate fields. This is difficult for even the best of supervisors, trying to guide the student through the maze of new journals, the comparative value of different Internet sites and the breadth of books in various languages from around the world. When the supervisor is inadequate or insecure, the result can be extremely negative. The supervisor may pretend knowledge of the field, or direct the student to an area with which he or she is familiar. Supervisors may suggest a joint publication, making use of the student's work to further their own prospects for promotion. In what is perhaps an illustration of a much larger problem of lack of recognition for junior academics, one woman in the group stated that a joint publication resulted in no benefit to her. Supervisors may opt out, and limit their contribution to correcting grammar and commenting on the font size in a process of withdrawal from the problem. The situation is often further compounded when the supervisor is male and the student is female.

The structural requirements of a PhD necessitate that the relationship continues over a number of years. Accordingly, there is potential for much to go wrong. Our stories show some of the ways this can happen, as well as instances where the mentoring role worked extremely well. However, given the current context, good (or even workable) relationships should be celebrated, so strong are the countervailing factors mitigating against such a process actually working effectively.

Our study has focused on the student perspective of the process, and has shared aspects of the lived research experience of some women. What got things going, as it were, was not usually an intellectual question, but often a strong emotion which was then named and given an intellectual voice: anger at being passed over, determination to prove that it could be done.

Intellectualizing the experience has been a positive means of coping with those deep, ambivalent emotions. The more we talked with women who had embarked on the PhD journey, the more we found that an emotional reason was at the core of their 'getting started' or sticking with their study. Thus, the place of the emotions in learning, in intellectualizing, in theorizing, seems to us to be crucial. Although we did not use the methodology of memory-work *per se* (Haug, 1987; Crawford *et al.*, 1990), we are sympathetic to that approach and see it as deepening those understandings of the doctoral research process that have emerged from our questionnaires, interviews and focus group discussions. Indeed, in reflecting upon our methodology we realize that we did not rely solely upon these strategies, but also drew on our own memories of conversations with some of the participants over years of journeying together. Memories of sharing a cup of coffee after a bad session with a supervisor when self-esteem felt at rock bottom, a celebratory drink after a grant was successful, a listening time after a particularly traumatic episode with a partner or the children, a struggle session as to how to make best use of data that took months to collect but seemed to be saying nothing. These memories of ours, the researchers, are as much part of the methodology as the actual questionnaires and recorded discussion. Allowing the data to tell a story that has broader significance than that embodied in individual highlights is our aim.

One of the components that we recognize as important is allowing the personal story to be seen as a valid part of understanding the doctoral journey; the way in which the experience of juggling commitments and opening one's mind to new ideas were all part of the personal fabric of undertaking a PhD. There is also the intermeshed emotional world of relating to one's partner, children, parents and possibly other family members, and the changing world of friends and fellow travellers.

In some ways these stories are ephemeral. The four years – or six, or ten – have flown and life has moved on. Memories of anger, of drudgery, of helplessness, of delight, fade over time. What may seem highly valuable in one's thirties may be perceived as less so in one's fifties. The personal challenge of seeing a task to completion recedes in value as new challenges arise. For this reason, the memories that the women bring are not a reflection of the experience itself. Rather, as those who have engaged in research using memory-work as a tool are wont to remind us, it is *the memory* itself which has value (as an object, a commodity), which can be gazed upon, reflected about, laughed at. It allows one to relive anger, pride, frustration and wonderment in the company of others who have also traversed that journey. But more than that, it gives permission for that object of the memory to be a means by which further understanding of one's motives, one's dreams and one's aspirations may be understood as social items, items that are interrelated with other simultaneous journeys.

Charting new waters

Is change occurring in the tertiary education sector? Despite the many difficulties experienced by overworked academics, there are subtle transformations taking place in the institution itself. Part of the reason is the increasing number of women engaged in a wide range of research, and the increasing number of women who are now supervisors. Structures, support systems, the nature of research topics, are always fluid, even although at times they look as if they are set in concrete. Their essential fluidity arises from their socially constructed nature (Berger and Luckmann, 1972). From a policy-making perspective, one might question the nature of the 'rite of passage' demanded by academia, when the rite itself generates so much angst. There is something of value, and it is that which we need to retain. As more women are systematically integrated into higher education it is not just their voice that will make a difference; it is not just the measurable items of research that may pertain to women that may increase; rather it is the nature of higher education itself that will slowly change.

After taking the plunge and riding the waves, the ocean not merely sustains but empowers. We who have gone through this rite of passage inevitably bring changes to the doctoral process. We are committed to enhancing professional practice as well as knowledge. Despite the established codes and hierarchies of academia of which the PhD is a powerful manifestation, there are uncharted waters in which these rules do not apply. It is in these waters that our collaborative research has been nourished. We have come to realize that where open, honest and trusting relationships exist, new forms emerge that transcend individual achievement. Where the personal, emotional, multi-layered element of learning is recognized, validated and affirmed, then new insights and understandings of the doctoral process, its potentialities and pitfalls surface and, like the ripples, can be spread outwards in all directions. It is for others to respond and judge the value of this learning, but we believe that the emancipatory moments that we each uniquely experienced can become part of a collective experience.

[1]An original version of this chapter was published in the proceedings of *Winds of Change: Women and the Culture of Universities* International Conference, July, 1998, UTS, Sydney.

References

Arnold, R. (1997) The theory and principles of psychodynamic pedagogy. *Forum of Education*, **49**(2), 21–33.

Berger, P. L. and Luckmann, T. (1972) *The Social Construction of Reality: A Treatise in the Sociology of Knowledge*. Ringwood: Penguin.

Craig, J. E. and Spear, N. (1982) Rational actors, group processes and the development of educational system. In *The Sociology of Educational Expansion* (M. Archer, ed.), p. 14. London: Sage.

Crawford, J., Kippax, S., Onyx, J., Gault, U. and Benton, P. (1990) Women theorising their experiences of anger: a study using memory-work. *Australian Psychologist*, **25**(3), 333–350.

Elbaz-Luwisch, F. (1997) Narrative research: political issues and implications. *Teaching and Teacher Education*, **3**(1), 75–83.

Evans, B. L. (1998) Golden jubilee for Australian PhDs. *Campus Review*, Special Report, April 1–7, p. 13.

Haug, F. (1987) *Female Sexualization: A Collective Work of Memory*. London: Verso.

Hayes, E. and Flannery, D. D. (1997) Narratives of adult women's learning in higher education: insights from graduate research. *Initiatives*, **58**(2), 61–80.

LePage, P. and Flowers, D. (1995) Whose personal stories are published in educational journals? Investigating presumptions about women's subjectivity in academic discourse. *Initiatives*, **57**(1), 41–54.

Neumann, A. (ed.) (1997) *Learning From Our Lives: Women, Research and Autobiography in Education*. New York: Teachers' College Press.

Spendiff, A. (1992) Learning brings us together: the meaning of feminist adult education. In *Working and Learning Together for Change* (C. Biott and J. Nias, eds), pp. 109–129. Buckingham: Open University Press.

8

Whose show is it? The contradictions of collaboration

Hilary Byrne-Armstrong

Introduction

Notions such as cooperation, collaboration or participation evoke powerful ideals for those people who are attracted to qualitative research because of the perceived ethical issues of quantitative research; issues people see as produced by the assumption that the researcher can be totally impartial and make observations to come up with truths that are beyond contamination from human perspectives.[1] Co-researching *with* people rather than *on* them (Reason and Rowan, 1981) is a catch phrase used to imply research that is designed to challenge these seemingly oppressive practices of quantitative research. However, even these allegedly more ethical practices have their limitations. In this chapter I explore collaboration in research from the viewpoint that 'everything is dangerous' (Foucault, 1983).

Many ideas in qualitative research emerged out of the influence of liberal humanism on learning and research. Humanism centred the human subject as the originator of research and knowledge (rather than God), because human beings have the ability to act in the world and to be objective and impartial about their actions. Liberal humanism challenged the notion that human beings could be totally impartial. It injected the personal and subjective back into the research arena under the rubric of qualitative research (see Reason and Rowan, 1981). The researcher was no longer considered able to be impartial, and the researched were no longer inanimate objects but people who could join in the research as active participants. Consequently, we as practitioners became *co*-learners with students, *co*-researching with clients and *co*-authoring with colleagues. The prefix 'co-' became as popular in radical/experiential learning and qualitative research as the 'post-' prefix has in contemporary philosophy!

I hasten to say that I am not against these things (this book provides a concrete example). What I do want to do is 'sing up'[2] some experiences that I have had as a co-researcher which have led me to question collaborative research practices and consequently to modify my own. I want to critique aspects of the influence of liberal humanism in this area, because I think that oversimplified prescriptions embedded in notions such as 'co-research' reinforce the very thing they were aiming to address, the imbalance of power found in much quantitative research. Sentimentalizing co-learning and co-research as processes with equality hides the inevitable power differences that exist between people who engage in research, learning, or any activity, for that matter. Instead of being visible and overt, power becomes invisible and covert, hidden behind layers of paternalism and what I have called elsewhere a 'tyranny of niceness' (Byrne-Armstrong, 1999). This is what I explore in this chapter. I use three anecdotes from my researching experience that, when linked together, illustrate the existence of power differences as well as suggesting a pathway through the web of power–knowledge relationships that entangles qualitative research processes. First, I will recount the narratives.

Narrative One

I had returned to University as a mature-aged student in a Graduate Diploma programme focusing on adult education principles. In the major work for my final year, I undertook a project situated in qualitative research methodologies. I was an excited new researcher who, coming from the health sciences (where research was dominated by the shadow of the bell curve), was delighted to embrace methods for research that actually involved talking to people and listening to their experience and making sense of it rather than dismissing it as 'anecdotal' and therefore not valid.

I situated myself within research that was viewed as a 'reciprocal and relational process in which co-researchers are actively contributing to the design, content and method of the process' (Byrne-Armstrong, 1994, p. 60). The method I chose was participatory action research (PAR) (Reason and Rowan, 1981). The participants and I met in a group to air our shared interest and concerns, reflect on our research goals, and design interventions to achieve them. In each subsequent research meeting, we reflected on our progress and designed further interventions. Informing this research was 'constructivism', a view of knowledge that proposes that there is no truth to be found 'out there'. Truth emerges from people relating and negotiating meanings. The research report included, therefore, not only *what* we achieved in terms of learning, but also *how* we achieved it through the negotiations that we carried out along the way.

I was interested in the health care relationship as a learning relationship, and the influence people's learning styles might have on this relationship. My idea was that knowing our own and others' learning styles might facilitate learning and communication in health education. I gathered some interested colleagues in the health area and asked them to join me as co-researchers. Initially, we spent several sessions exploring qualitative research processes and getting to know each other. To begin the research process, we agreed to identify our own learning styles. It was at this point that one of my colleagues said, 'This is no different from mainstream research. I have a guinea-pig feeling when you suggest we identify our learning styles – if I feel like this, what do you think our clients will feel?'.[3]

Outwardly I nodded sympathetically, inwardly I felt it as a despairing moment. Where was this comment coming from? How was it that my co-researcher still felt this way after the ethical issues and the differences between qualitative research and quantitative research processes had been so thoroughly aired?

Narrative Two

Some years passed and this intrepid researcher undertook yet another stage in her learning ('women can never be educated enough') and research. In my exploration of experiential learning, I became fascinated by the way people applied a training model called the experiential learning cycle in training sessions. The experiential learning cycle was a model developed by Kolb (1984) based on the way people learn through problem-solving. Kolb proposed that people used a process of acting, experiencing, reflecting and making sense to solve problems. He suggested that these four brain activities did not occur in any order; they were simultaneous and continuous. In other words, Kolb was careful to emphasize that this process was not linear, sequential, necessarily rational, or prescriptive. However, in my observation of trainers using Kolb's work, I was struck by the way that it was used prescriptively and sequentially. Training sessions were designed around the four aspects, the idea being that if people sequentially experienced each function on the cycle they would have learnt 'how to learn'. My suspicion was that learning was not neat and ordered, as the application of these methods would suggest. Learning was a messy and diffuse process.

I designed a research project for a Masters thesis to explore for myself how the four so-called brain functions were expressed in learning. I proposed a collaborative project in which I brought together a group of people who were learning a new form of psychotherapeutic practice. We agreed that we would use a variety of processes to reflect on how we learned, as we learned (Byrne-Armstrong, 1994). While I framed the project as collaborative, I was aware that it was only partially collaborative in that I was attaining a higher degree and my co-researchers were not. I did not mention this issue. However, one of my co-researchers was sharper than I was! At a group meeting that person said, 'Why, if this is co-research and fully collaborative, don't we all get a Masters degree?'.

This conflict of interest (and I would be more frank about the limitations of collaboration now) muddied the waters of the research, and had consequences later on. After a session where I attempted to pull together the meanings for my thesis, the group rebelled and asked me to complete it on my own. Only two of them wanted to read drafts, and two the final copy.

Narrative Three

The next incident emerged from yet another piece of work (this researcher is a slow learner!). I had initiated a project of reconciliation/mediation involving a cross-cultural group. I was clearer about power. I said that although I was the initiator, which gave me a different position in the group (in that I had chosen the research and brought the group together), this was a piece of co-research. My co-researchers were relieved that I had voiced this sentiment and satisfied with the paradox that this position entailed ... until it came time to finish the research. They complained. 'Not only do you initiate and select the group, but you also have the power to pull the plug', one participant said.

After some time, these three narratives connected in my mind. I decided to explore the (my) assumptions about collaborative forms of research. My first question led me to research the philosophical roots of the forms of research in which I was engaged. As stated earlier, research processes are mostly embedded in humanism, which situates human subjects and their experiences as the starting point for knowledge because of their unique ability to objectify or distance themselves from the subjects of their scrutiny. Collaboration within qualitative research implies a challenge to this separation of the subject and object. In fact it challenges the very notion that it is possible to separate subject and object, and argues for research in which there is a more conscious joining together of subject and object, researcher and researched.

However, traces of positivist research are still present in qualitative research. First, the subject/object opposition still frames qualitative research, in that 'rigour' in qualitative research is the ability to be objective while still being engaged. The rhetoric about this can be found in techniques for 'bracketing' as in phenomenological research (Sass, 1990), 'self-reflexivity' in feminist research (Stanley, 1990) or in the 'subjective objectivity' of Reason and Rowan (1981). The issue is that these processes still uphold objectivity because of the connection between objectivity and truth, which leads to my second point. Objectivity is glorified in the name of 'truth'. Human beings' ability to be objective is thought to be the reason that they have access to the truth. Education (including research) is the way that people learn objectivity, and therefore is the pathway to truth. The philosophical belief is that, once educated, truth will be found, and people will liberate themselves and create a civil society, '... and the result will be wholesome, bathed in sunshine, smelling of hay, cider with Rosie, entirely free from red-back or funnel-web spiders' (Newman, 1994, p. 20).

Participatory action research is one such formula for realizing human potential. Through the participatory research process, individual consciousness is raised, promoting transformation and liberating the 'true' and civil nature of human beings. My difficulty is that in this individualistic and truth-seeking activity, social positioning, cultural differences and power relationships remain invisible or buried, ironically, in the name of equality, collaboration. Who determines the truth, and whose interest it serves, is hidden. An example occurs in the research narratives above, where the implicit interests (of the initiator and her context) served by the research were disguised in the idealistic notion of collaboration. I was the one writing the research document and the one who gained a degree. My group asked why, if it was collaborative, didn't all of us get a degree?

Can there ever be full collaboration or participation when groups are made up of people with a complexity of interests and agendas? I don't think so. Collaboration gets 'totalised' (Foucault, 1977) by the sentimentality of the liberal humanist ideal. The fact that collaboration is a paradox is hidden under the weight of humanism's ideals and sentiment (it's too 'nice' to contest, says Newman, 1994). Simple examples of the paradoxical nature of collaboration can be found in the narratives above.

- Narrative One: It was my agenda to explore learning styles, not the group's agenda. Although a collaborative group may be formed, the questions and topics in any research belong to a certain agenda that serves the interests of the researcher.

- Narrative Two: I received the degree. The research always serves the interests of some people more than others. These can be funding bodies, grants committees, or, as in this case, the individual working towards a degree.
- Narrative Three: Although people with common interests are brought together in the name of collaborating to talk about and design interventions around common concerns, one person initiates the research as well as calls a halt to it. This action is a power-full and non-collaborative act.

In most cases, power differences in collaborative research processes are not explicit. It is important to regard research as a 'way of seeing' that serves certain people's interests; in the cases described in the narratives, the interests were mine. However, it is also true that collaborative research processes can have a ripple effect on the lives of others. Following the research group mentioned in the second incident, all members of the group continued their education (in very different directions, both informal and formal), and three of the five went on to higher degrees.

I learned from these experiences to be open and 'up front' about power issues from the beginning. But I do not think that this is enough. Although collaborative methodologies emphasize the constructed nature of knowledge, embedded as they are in liberal humanist thought, they remain focused on the human subject and her/his interactions. Collaborative methodologies give little attention to the assumptions (e.g. the subject/object opposition and the power of 'truth') that frame their practices in the first place. While we keep focusing on individual human subjects (for example, arguing about how objective and subjective we should be), we fail to address the language games and social practices that create us as separate individuals in the first place. To address these we could ask questions like, 'What is the history of the methods that separate people into subjects and objects?', 'What is the history that shapes some people as objects?', 'How do these methods affect people?'.

Changing directions . . .

My conclusion (for the moment) is that collaboration can occur only if we move away from researching to find truth, whether it is on people (positivism), or with people (co-research), and move towards joining with people in conversation to examine the taken-for-granted assumptions and practices informing any research context. This is because my present position is that language does not represent the world. Our view of the world comes from the meanings (narratives) we make of our experience. In other words, we don't just story the world, we story ourselves in a world (Michelfelder and Palmer, 1989). This position heralds a shift of research focus from the human subject as meaning-maker to the meanings/narratives themselves. My interest is in how these meanings are produced and re-produced and their influence on the relationships and social practices in any context; a change of emphasis from methods that focus on individual meanings to methods that focus on the cultural narratives and their influence on our lives.

For example, in Narrative One, the cultural narrative informing the research was the medical discourse. This is a set of social practices and language games that have a history and a particular way of thinking about 'health'. The practices of the medical discourse include positioning the responsibility of our health with an expert doctor or health professional, and positioning medical knowledge formulated through scientific means as the only true knowledge about health. Other knowledge, such as the patient's personal experience, is considered not valid knowledge and is silenced. These are two examples showing how people and knowledge are positioned in power relationships within a cultural narrative.

In the above example, I have demonstrated a central practice of this form of research. I have positioned (in language) the medical discourse as separate from the co-researchers. In other words, I have externalized[4] it. Once we have positioned ourselves in this way, we can co-research our experiences of the medical discourse in order to examine the ways that it does and does not encourage self-responsibility and learning in the face of illness. A question I would now ask people in this piece of research is: how do medical 'social practices' such as the ones described above influence the health care relationship, and is this helpful to health, to our body? In the second narrative, I would examine the educational discourse and its methods, such as learning style tests, to find out the influence these tests have on people as learners. In the third narrative, I would externalize discourses of racism and power and ask how they were being played out in the research context as well as in people's lives, and the effect on their self-determination. This process of joining together to co-research the dominant practices shaping our lives is what I am now calling collaboration.

My current research practice is a weaving together of hermeneutics, in that it is interpretive (exploring how we make one interpretation and not another), and it is poststructuralist, in that it is not seeking a final truth/ interpretation. In other words, I have developed a narrative analysis with a Foucauldian twist. I will now briefly discuss how I came to weave together these two methodologies.[5]

Hermeneutics is an interpretive method that has been described as 'just one example of an everyday process through which people make sense of their worlds' (Rowan, 1981, p. 132). It heralds for me a step away from researching with people to researching the narratives that people use to make sense of their world. The goal of hermeneutics as I am defining it is to discover the underlying meaning present in language and text (text can be image and movement) through a cooperative process. Hermeneutics acknowledges that shared meanings are constituted in culture, language and symbols, but claims that these can be refined and interpreted to uncover an underlying meaning. Furthermore, hermeneutics recognizes that we are historical beings situated in a place at a point of time in a particular culture. Therefore, people's narratives are situated in time and place. This means that any interpretation will depend on when and where it was formed. In other words, people's assumptions and preconceptions as writers, speakers or researchers are culturally and historically bound, and the underlying meaning will reflect this situatedness.

Narrative One illustrated this phenomenon. We live in the soup of mainstream research practices. No matter how ethical or collaborative we are in qualitative research processes, the power of the mainstream narrative of research at this point of history will be present and will, to some extent, shape our research. This situatedness presents both the pathway to recognizing that all knowledge is grounded in human relationships (and is therefore a challenge to mainstream research processes that imply that knowledge is abstract and universal) and my point of departure from hermeneutics, because of its belief in a universal truth.

Hermeneutics implies a universal truth when it 'reach(es) for an interpretation which is intersubjectively valid for all people who share the same world at a given time in history' (Rowan, 1981, p. 133). This insistence on the presence of an interpretation, valid for all people, is my point of departure from hermeneutics. As soon as there is an attempt to homogenize different viewpoints, meanings or experiences into thematic/universal interpretations, the collaborative process changes to a colonizing process. If one assumes that life and human beings are complex, different and diverse, any collaboration must include multiple voices rather than a single voice. Therefore, any search for a single answer or truth will silence voices, and will perpetuate to some extent what many of us most want to challenge about mainstream research processes.

My thinking and practice therefore moved one step further in the 'turn towards language' (Byrne-Armstrong, 1999), not to find deeper meanings and truth, but to look for multiple interpretations.[6] Engaging in what Geertz (1983, p. 34) called 'an elaborate venture into thick description', the method I am exploring both as a researcher and teacher analyses the self-narratives in any context, treating them as expressions of social practices that produce and are produced by prevailing (dominant) cultural narratives (e.g. the three examples earlier were medical, education and racist discourses). The exploration occurs *in situ* (at the local level of practice), therefore incorporating the narratives of others, and in this sense is collaborative and hermeneutic. However, in the sense that the aim is not to find a shared, deeper meaning or generalizable truth, but to sing up many truths/narratives, it is poststructuralist.

In summary, I realize that in saying my work is both hermeneutic and poststructuralist, I am combining two contested streams of Western thought.[7] Both streams agree that language is in charge of us. However, one stream seeks to strengthen the movement towards unity and tradition by emphasizing the authority and truth in/of texts. The other emphasizes the slipperiness of language and text, questioning the concept of meaning itself. Meanings are therefore played with and the text interpreted many times, producing a multiplicity and plurality of interpretations, or narratives. A collaboration, therefore, is expressed in multiple voices rather than ending up as a single voice. However, the aim of the work is not only to provide a space for multiple voices to be heard, but also to make visible a political process. In the presence of multiple voices, one can demonstrate the power difference among voices (the Foucauldian aspect of the analysis). Some voices (knowledges) are silenced and other voices and knowledges dominate the airwaves. This power difference is the impetus for the political aspect of this work.

This researcher considers that a research process can be collaborative only if the co-researchers turn their collective attention away from the search for a consensus of understanding and turn it to asking why or where this notion comes from in the first place. If, in the face of funding bodies and boards of faceless examiners, consensus is still considered the only way forward, then co-researchers should ask, 'In this consensus, what voices are being silenced, what knowledge is being rendered unspeakable?'. Questions such as this challenge the dominant rhetoric of research, which would have us believe that rigorous research of any kind must reduce the complexity of human lives to universal themes/generalizations through common understandings and consensus.

My changing interpretations of the narratives recounted in this chapter led me from being an enthusiastic humanist inquirer searching with people for truth and meaning, to a bewildered sense of the collaborative research process, and then a dawning cynicism. 'Collaboration' now means to me just another method that serves a dominant narrative that promotes divisive methods in the name of a universal truth. Homogenizing difference into generalized themes is not collaboration but colonization. Not only does it silence voices, it also disguises power. The philosophical position that I now hold is that there is no single truth to be found, just more interpretations. The interpretation we call the truth is the one that is attached to power (in research, the power is usually associated with researcher, or with the organization providing the finance). No matter how collaborative a process is, the connection between power and knowledge will determine the truth. Furthermore, as Foucault said, 'since the hidden meaning is not the final truth about what is going on, finding it is not necessarily liberating; in fact it can lead away from the kind of understanding which might help the actors resist the current practices of domination' (Foucault, 1983, p. 124). Currently I am interested in research processes that assist in the development of the sorts of understanding that Foucault implies. I have journeyed away from co-research with people to co-research (with or without people) with the collective interpretations and narratives that constitute our lives.

[1] There are many excellent texts on the limitations of quantitative research especially in feminist literature, e.g. Nicholson (1990), Stanley (1990), Reinharz (1992). See also Reason and Rowan (1981).

[2] I am using 'sing up' metaphorically to evoke the notion that our language and meaning-making are processes that emerge with language, constructs of how we view the world. It is also a reference to the Aboriginal notion of singing the land.

[3] Interestingly, we never did get to the point of working with clients on this issue.

[4] To 'externalize' the medical discourse means to position it in language as a 'thing' that is separate from people. By positioning themselves within language in this way, people can then view themselves as distinct from it and as having choices about when to follow it and when to resist.

[5] For a fuller discussion of my current methodologies, see Byrne-Armstrong (1999).

[6] The beginning of my poststructuralist interests.

[7] An excellent book on this argument is *Dialogue and Deconstruction: the Gadamer–Derrida Encounter* (Michelfelder and Palmer, 1989).

References

Byrne-Armstrong, H. (1994) Spinning the threads of Indira's net: reflexivity in action. MSc (Hons) thesis, University of Western Sydney, Hawkesbury, NSW, Australia.

Byrne-Armstrong, H. (1999) Dead certainties and local knowledge: poststructuralism, conflict and narrative practices in radical/experiential education. PhD thesis, University of Western Sydney, Hawkesbury, NSW, Australia.

Foucault, M. (1977) *Discipline and Punish: The Birth of a Prison*. London: Peregrine Books.

Foucault, M. (1983) Afterword: the subject and power. In *Michel Foucault: Beyond Structuralism and Hermeneutics* (H. Dreyfus and P. Rabinow, eds), 2nd edn, pp. 208–226. Chicago: University of Chicago Press.

Geertz, C. (1983) *Local Knowledge: Further Essays in Interpretive Anthropology*. London: Fontana Press.

Kolb, D. (1984) *Experiential Learning*. Englewood Cliffs: Prentice Hall.

Michelfelder, D. and Palmer, R. (1989) *Dialogue and Deconstruction: The Gadamer–Derrida Encounter*. New York: State University of New York Press.

Newman, M. (1994) *Defining the Enemy*. Sydney: Victor Stuart.

Nicholson, L. (1990) *Feminism Postmodernism*. New York: Routledge.

Reason, P. and Rowan, J. (eds) (1981) *Human Inquiry: A Sourcebook of New Paradigm Research*. London: John Wiley & Sons.

Reinharz, S. (1992) *Feminist Methods in Social Research*. Oxford: Oxford University Press.

Rowan, J. (1981) A dialectical paradigm for research. In *Human Inquiry: A Sourcebook of New Paradigm Research* (P. Reason and J. Rowan, eds), pp. 93–112. London: John Wiley & Sons.

Sass, L. (1990) Humanism and hermeneutics. In *Hermeneutics and Psychological Theory: Interpretative Perspectives on Personality, Psychotherapy and Psychopathology* (S. Messer, L. Sass and R. Woolfolk, eds), pp. 222–271. London: Rutgers University Press.

Stanley, L. (ed.) (1990) *Feminist Praxis: Research and Epistemology*. London: Routledge.

9

Playing in the 'mud' of government

Virginia Kaufman Hall

When you plant a lettuce, if it does not grow well, you don't blame the lettuce. You look for reasons it is not doing well. It may need fertilizer, or more water, or less sun. You never blame the lettuce . . .

No blame, no reasoning, no argument, just understanding.

If you understand and you show that you understand, you can love, and the situation will change. (Thich Nhat Hahn, 1991)[1]

Just as the farmer must balance life-giving elements, so must good government policy-makers balance competing interests to develop the desired outcomes. In my work as a social research consultant, I undertake needs analysis, project management, community development and evaluations for all levels of government. As a qualitative researcher, I strive to understand and identify what makes effective government policies and programmes. My 'passion' is social justice and equity. Most of my work involves applying qualitative research skills to projects where my role is often to tell the stories of those whose voices are rarely heard in places of power.

We research to understand; through understanding we care, and because we care we work at changing situations where people are restricted in their capacity to grow. A wise farmer watches the lettuce crop closely. A wise policy-maker uses qualitative research to detail evidence of what works and what doesn't.

This chapter is my story about the realities of working as a research consultant for government; it is about the *messy parts* and *critical moments* of playing in the mud. The nitty-gritty realities of hard politics compete against many vested interests and lobby groups, so that social justice does not always score a win.

Why are qualitative research tools valuable when applied to policy and programme development? Based upon my five years researching for government, I explore how public policy and programme development can be influenced through using qualitative research skills. Here is a 'snapshot' of qualitative research methodology in the public sector that may well be useful if you wonder what jobs you can attract with research skills among your qualifications.

Government policy-makers and programme evaluators use qualitative research skills: scoping or mapping, in-depth inquiry into complex situations, consultation, bottom-up policy development recommendations, social analysis, and extracting major issues from story-telling. Stories are powerful when they are collected from people whose voices may not normally be heard by policy-makers, as in the *Bringing Them Home* report of the 'stolen children' (National Inquiry into the Separation of Aboriginal and Torres Strait Islander Children from their Families, 1997).

What were the influences and critical moments that led to my career in social research?

Communities of practice

Having been a teenager in the 1960s, raised as a social activist during the cold war years, I hold a strong belief in the Buddhist concept of 'right livelihood', and I have faith that appropriate answers lie within *communities of people*. Techniques and processes to activate 'communities of practice' are strengthened by experience. This experiential learning has come through raising three children to adults with the support of a civil community and our extended 'non-kin' family.

Grounded feminism

While designing education and training programmes for women returning to the workforce, I learned grounded feminist theory.[2] I was enriched by a definition from a young Cypriot woman, Helen:

> *What's good for women and children is good for everyone.*

This definition also works for social justice.

I explored the concept of accelerating social justice into the workplace through my PhD thesis (Kaufman Hall, 1996[3]) by building upon what others had already discovered. The processes of interviewing and of facilitating thirteen workshops with the twelve co-researchers included in the thesis identified best practice in social justice workplace activism and life–work balance. I came to understand more about how the real world works by this research, writing and reflecting to make meaning out of it all so it may be useful to others inquiring into whether what we do at work determines how we and others experience the world.

Cooperative inquiry

Through teaching and supervising for five years and researching social ecology over twelve years, I learned the practice of cooperative inquiry in which I apply my conflict resolution, facilitation, mediation and change-agent skills. I work as a storyteller, collecting stories from people so they are heard by the policy-makers. I often use their words to ground the meta-analysis, identifying the policy initiative that can make a difference.

Action learning

When I arrived in the Australian capital I had just completed six years' immersion in gaining a PhD while working full time. At 49 years, the move was designed as an opportunity to launch into my fifth career[4] – this time as a research consultant. It was not an entirely new venture. I had been operating as a 'change/research consultant' for over five years in research and community development projects.

My considerable research experience and theoretical knowledge required an open mind and respectful curiosity. This is how I see qualitative research as an experience that is different from quantitative or secondary data research. In the best projects, it means researchers are on site in the research situation. That is the bit I love; experiencing the context of where people live and work is very different from simply gathering demographic and purely statistical data (which may also be useful).

'Action learning' in my context is *learning by doing* the fieldwork *and* making sense of it for the policy-makers.

Government as client – tensions in the role

In the last decade of the twentieth century, most first world governments moved to outsource many internal functions. Thus needs analyses, programme management, community development and evaluations are now regularly outsourced. Whatever ideologies we might hold about the legitimacy of moving functions out of the public sector, the strategy furnishes opportunities for qualitative researchers to use their multiple methodological skills to provide many of these functions.

Many bureaucratic jobs inside government involve using research and analysis skills. Bureaucrats collect data and information, then carefully file the data that tell part of the story. The 'creative bit' comes when applying one's skills to make sense of it all by writing reports, analysing outcomes and occasionally proposing policy directions. Practically, this means that qualitative research skills can be applied to many public sector or industry careers, no matter what the job title. These qualitative research skills are invaluable to any development work involving strategic planning, industry and community business plans and social analysis. However, government advertisements do not immediately reveal this aspect. The job descriptions often do not state that *research* skills are required.

Inquiry into government language – what does it mean?

The ability to work with the language and concepts of economics helps with being heard in an economic rationalist climate. A qualitative researcher must be able to tell the story revealed by statistics, using other specialists' language, in order to succeed and be accepted as 'legitimate'. In this sense a researcher's language in reports must often reflect the 'tribal' language and organizational culture of the particular government client. I have *not* found an over-arching acceptance of qualitative research terminology and concepts among government bureaucrats. Most likely their individual backgrounds and education do not encompass qualitative research. Educating this audience can be time-consuming and frustrating, but is critical to getting the research accepted. Perhaps, in reality, I get more education as I discover the culture and language of different government departments.

Matching language is critical in fulfilling requirements for the Government's tendering process for research contracts. There are special meanings of terms; every brief advises consultants to seek clarification if a phrase is confusing.

Reality itself can be challenged by government. Look at this example of the absurdity of language endeavouring to reconstruct reality, in legislation by the Australian Government in Section 165-55 of *A New Tax System* (1999) allowing the Tax Commissioner to:

> ... *treat a particular event that actually happened as not having happened* ...
> *{and to} treat a particular event that did not actually happen as having happened and if appropriate treat the event as having happened at a particular time and treat a particular event that actually happened as having involved particular action by a particular entity whether or not the event actually involved any action by that entity.*

Does this contextual view of reality amount to postmodernism in legislation?

Negotiating the structural barrier of economic rationalism? (or supporting due process within government to demonstrate that funding has been spent as parliament intended)

Many observers of Australian government have commented that an economic rationalist approach to policy development has supplanted virtually all competing perspectives, and is now entrenched (Pusey, 1991). Anyone who wants to be taken seriously within government circles has adopted the language and practice of economic rationalism. What does this view of reality mean to those wanting to pursue qualitative research within an economic rationalist climate and culture?

Fortunately, qualitative researchers' competence in multiple methodologies means that we can integrate useful and appropriate methodologies in our inquiries. If researchers are hired by government (either as consultants or employees), then government as a primarily political institution wants to demonstrate effective and strong policies and programmes.

Early in 1999, I interviewed five managers of research and evaluation, policy development and business development sections from five different Commonwealth Government departments (individual positions are not identified, to preserve anonymity). The interviews (from which the following quotations come) focused specifically on how government uses qualitative research.

One senior manager summed it up as follows:

> *The most powerful research for government is to find out what we need to quantify. Once the area of inquiry is identified, then the statistics provide the 'facts' politicians need and people want to hear. However, statistics have to be*

accurately targeted to be effective. The strongest process to get a change of policy through the bureaucracy is to use a combination of methodologies.

Coming from an experienced researcher, this statement describes the process of triangulation: using multiple methods to validate data. In these cases quantitative research provides the bones; qualitative research fleshes it out with explanatory stories, social impact experiences, expected and unexpected spin-offs and useful information for drafting possible future policy initiatives. Government then uses this research to justify what it wants to do.

It was the view of two interviewees that politicians and some public servant executives are *afraid* of qualitative research:

Politicians and senior bureaucrats like numbers because they can use them. Quantitative research badly done can still be quoted.

This advice may also serve as the qualitative researcher's guide to working within a climate of economic rationalism. It is easier to state a research result as 'Eighty per cent of Australian employers find ...'. Figures sound stronger than a report that 'there was an overwhelming feeling that ...'. Bureaucrats (and politicians) are often uncomfortable with what seems to them to be 'soft' or 'vague' language in a research report.

Oscar Wilde defined a cynic as a '... man who knows the price of everything and the value of nothing' (*Oxford Dictionary of Quotations*, 1985). Quantitative research in government terms (rightly) considers the price and output of policy as being very important. Qualitative research (among other factors) presents the outcomes, value and the cost of policies revealed in stories from the 'muddy' and often untidy playground of life.

Research as a tool for change (so we not only know the price of everything, but the cost and the value of what was purchased)

Four of the five public servants interviewed use research as a tool for change. In fact, unless change is a likely outcome, they see no point in doing the research. One applies twenty years' experience to identifying the processes necessary for research to bring about change and/or benchmark effective practice. Rather than agonize about whether a qualitative or quantitative approach is preferable, they pragmatically blend the two. The combined approach allows research and evaluation sections in government to identify the questions to ask in a (follow-up) quantitative survey. Applying the two approaches in reverse allows for qualitative methods to explore what will make the difference; quantitative data identifies the *dimensions* of a problem area.

Statistics are useful to set the frame for the research area. If researchers then want to find out *how* to make a difference, story-telling methodologies are applied for revealing detail. As all effective research poses further questions, the budget implications of further research are prioritized. If fieldwork is necessary the cost increases; if secondary data are used the cost decreases.

Once the research area is defined, qualitative methodology is adapted to explore and inquire into identifying areas of change. If policies are to be appropriate and relevant for community groups, I apply a sound practice of respectful inquiry.

My working definition of qualitative research

Taking into account the preceding contextual descriptions, here is my working definition of qualitative research:

> *It is a collection of processes useful for inquiry and exploration of stakeholder-driven interests and change.*

I describe it as a process of uncovering '*Human Centred Solutions*' – the name of my consultancy. To me, qualitative also means 'quality' research. Multiple inquiry processes serve to reveal qualities within the people targeted in the research scope. An ideal outcome (among many) is to strengthen the communities of practice and mutuality of interests as well as the individuals participating in it.

Principles of respectful inquiry

I am always conscious that research with people means we are telling others' stories. I conduct research by first facilitating the discovery of people's stories and then being the storyteller (as the report writer). It is essential to underpin both the collection and the telling of the narrative with three principles:

- *Conscious contextuality*. No man, woman or group is an island. Our culture, environment and life story serve to construct our daily experience(s).
- *Meetings with people as a 'sacred encounter'*. This Jewish concept (Dowrick, in Wilson, 2000) strengthens the idea that if I respect the experiences of those with whom I am researching, we can explore together ways of finding approaches to change and development that are identified by them as beneficial. This is a familiar conflict-resolution concept, which leads to the third principle:
- *Working together to identify human-centred solutions*. Researching with rather than 'on' people (Reason, 1994), we work together to uncover the story. Research leads to identifying areas for change and possible solutions, thus writing a new story. What that change is and how it is done lies within the people affected. This principle is vitally important.

Living is work and work is living[5]

How do I make a living out of what I love to do? I am still refining the answer to that question. The following reflections share a few lessons learned, and identify ongoing tensions and 'messy' moments. I have come to recognize that these tensions are part of the nature of qualitative researching. You will seldom find them in textbooks on the subject. The terrain of fieldwork includes the inevitability of getting 'messy' while playing in the mud.

The tension between getting the job done on time and working with professional and ethical principles of practice

Projects have limited timelines and budgets. In initial proposals, I work at communicating (or selling) ethical practice as political insurance. This means that I work *with* the participants to find out what are important issues in the project, and with whom; then the process includes pragmatic risk management.

There is rarely time for full consultation allowing developmental input from the target groups. As with most consultancy arrangements, initial research (to write the proposal, expression of interest, or request for tender) is done in one's unpaid time.

Muddy learning

With every project I learn more. Working on the ground means I collect mud between my toes and dust in my hair, symbolically taking a little bit of the research group's country with me. By working together we learn *about* each other. Whether this extends to learning *from* each other depends upon the nature of the relationships and the level of trust.

Even the most successful projects reveal new areas for exploration and more appropriate ways of working with specific groups. Learning is often a conscious outcome for qualitative researchers, who research to learn and understand. As people involved in a learning process, we also learn about ourselves.

The following story and learning about my research practice shows how the research principles of conscious contextuality, sacred encounters and identifying *human-centred solutions* work in my practice, even in muddy field work.

Project story – nurturing nature

I managed the National Breastfeeding Education Promotion 1998, the first ever funded by the Commonwealth Department of Health. Nursing Mothers Association of Australia, the peak non-government organization (NGO) on breastfeeding, won the tender. I worked with a team of dedicated and professional unpaid volunteers as well as four paid project officers and a specialist social marketing company. The team worked with an advisory group comprising academics, health professionals and the Commonwealth Government. Everyone involved had a passionate interest in the success of the project. The aim was to inform and support families regarding breastfeeding, and was especially directed at difficult-to-reach demographic segments (multi-ethnic families with languages other than English, low socio-economic group and indigenous families and young mothers).

Educational material reached new and expecting families in 70.2 per cent of Australia's postcode areas, mostly through volunteers. Evaluations revealed highly successful distribution and effectiveness, with a response rate of over 73 per cent on the evaluation surveys from the local volunteer groups and 38.8 per cent from participating health professionals. Evaluation showed that innovative forms of distribution, enriched by locally based volunteers including trained breastfeeding counsellors, positively supported new families. In writing the report (Kaufman Hall, 1998) I integrated statistical material with qualitative responses, strengthening and expanding our understanding of the impact.

A major strength of the project was that localized distribution of print material was done by people who knew their community. This local and sectoral distribution was much more effective than any anonymous broadcast centralized mail-out. Educational material was in most cases personally given to new families at times when they were preparing for a new baby in the family, e.g. at a baby goods shop or at pre-natal hospital visits. We built 'conscious contextuality' by project workers inquiring into specific ways to reach multi-ethnic, Aboriginal, young and low socio-economic group families. In this way they developed specialized and personal networks for distribution, and these relationships produced many lasting spin-offs. For families who *read* in languages other than English, translated material was specially developed, pre-tested by multi-lingual health workers.

Because distribution was locally based, people knew what worked in their communities. During the development phase of the material, local groups were informed about the project regularly through monthly newsletters and at all state conferences of the Nursing Mothers Association of Australia. Many local groups discussed their situation with project officers or with me, 'talking-up' community development strategies that were sustainable for volunteers.

New outlets for breastfeeding information included Family Support Services, maternity and baby shops, multiple ethnic centres, sports clubs, workplaces and youth centres. Remote areas were effectively covered, often using locally useful venues. For example, resident volunteers in Kambalda, a remote mining town in Western Australia, distributed leaflets, comics and promotional cards to mining sites, a gym, community areas, a school, a local bank and a toy library.

The comic material (designed with youth input) attracted interest from Aboriginal family groups and those using languages other than English. These groups were also enthusiastic about a low-literacy leaflet with many appealing pictures of babies and mothers and few words, demonstrating photographically how to breastfeed. Aboriginal health workers used this booklet with Aboriginal families. It was the most popular of all the material, depicting mothers and babies from different cultures including Aboriginal.

At the conclusion of the project, debriefing with the Commonwealth Department of Health identified some important lessons. The debriefing we wanted (all project officers in one place at the programme's conclusion) could not happen because of lack of travel funds. However, the government officer responsible for overseeing the project invited me to a formal afternoon tea, a 'sacred encounter', where we reflected upon some lessons learned:

- One important lesson was that if the (government minister or delegate) source of funding does not approve of the educational material, it does not get approved. That sounds obvious, but this reality was initially overridden by enthusiasm for innovative ways to get the message across. For example, to develop material for hard-to-reach groups, the social marketing agency prepared comics for young families, using street language. While focus group samples responded positively to the rough street language and the Advisory Group approved it, the Department of Health did not. The requirement to adjust language and image is understandable for nationally distributed material. Complaint letters to the minister could cause embarrassment should someone object to the use of taxpayers' funds for publishing what some might perceive as 'rude, crude language'.

• Numerous stakeholders mean a complex approval process. The NGO had experts who reviewed educational material before the advisory group and then the government. Final approval of text took many weeks as electronic drafts went around and around.

In debriefing with the Department of Health, we reflected that future project budgets would include face-to-face meetings to facilitate agreement with many stakeholders.[6]

Since then I have worked with the development of national educational material inside government departments. I have observed how carefully public servants review material before it is made public. In the national breastfeeding project we completed an extraordinary task over three months, from focus group input to publication. I observed from later projects that agencies (appropriately) invoice for additional time spent on required changes in design and text of printed material after receiving authorized revisions from a government client.

Learning from every project

While I deliver results of qualitative research on time and within budget, usually with extra 'value-for-money' benefits identified along the way, every project adds to my learning. The lessons learned emerge from a range of researching activities.

In my experience, informed Government or NGO clients and participants value the identification of issues emerging from qualitative research. Some appreciate the grounded detail of the stories. The most useful findings for departmental strategic managers and policy writers are the identification of themes guiding analysis of *why* clients' experiences occur and *why* things happen that they may not have anticipated: *conscious contextuality* in the analysis and recommendations.

Public consultation – can it be a sacred encounter?

There is a now a more heightened awareness of the need for governments to consult with affected parties or stakeholders. In some Australian Commonwealth Government departments, the writing template for ministerial briefings includes a compulsory question: '*Who was consulted in the preparation of this brief?*'.

Consultation, in this context, has at least two definitions:

- Collecting and presenting the views of those people likely to be or already affected by the policy direction.
- Being able to confirm that people have been informed about the policy, whether or not there has been an effective consultation process with time for feedback and cooperative policy development.

Taking time to consult

Although government departments rarely have the time to consult effectively, some make the best use of the resources available to them. Nationwide consultation by the Council for Aboriginal Reconciliation (CAR) resulted in a fully collaborative final document. I had the privilege of facilitating a session for Jackie Huggins in Canberra at the beginning of the national consultation process. Jackie, a high profile member of CAR, played a major role in the public consultation process and is also an author, academic and Aboriginal activist. A meeting such as this was a sacred encounter, where more than a hundred local people, including local elders and the State Minister for Education, sat on the floor listening to and telling their stories of connections and reconciliation.

In Australia, I have worked on a number of public participation consultations for various government departments. I check with local or specific interest groups to see how a policy or project might be perceived and/or experienced. Usually I facilitate meetings with the stakeholders. My experience has been that if people want to participate, they do so in a way that makes sure they are heard. An invitation is often interpreted by participants as an opportunity to be heard and have their point of view taken seriously. However, a facilitator needs to be prepared to mediate or intervene to ensure that quieter, introvert voices are heard amongst the more articulate, perhaps noisier participants.

Consultation unearths local history

I ran an environmental consultation of focus groups to test the plans and displays in a new nature reserve facility. Stakeholders included passionate land users with an historical connection to the area for over a hundred years. Although no longer resident, they embodied a great deal of knowledge and retained an emotional connection to the land. Inviting them to the consultation allowed further historical information to emerge. These stories, which were then included in visitors' information materials, might never have come to light without the consultation. Such an example of qualitative research 'value added benefit' is a bonus clients appreciate and may remember when selecting tenderers.

Consulting for risk management

Another lesson I have learned in consultation processes is the need to work with a situation where not all the participants are satisfied with the process. Anyone trained in mediation tries to work with agreements and expanding options. However, agreement with a delegate does not translate into agreement with all participants. The integrity of the qualitative research result sometimes means that there will be participative dissenters.

I work at obtaining clearly, *in writing*, agreement on the process for reporting on feedback from individuals. One way to do this is to discuss a process and write it up for agreement with an authorized client signature. (On one occasion where I confirmed the last step verbally but not in writing, in a mixed group of industry, agencies and government, one group did not want to be identified as a source of the reported input.)

In my experience, it is not unusual for oral comments to be experienced as confrontational when reported in *written* form. For this reason I always present a draft report for input and adaptation, and encourage a round table meeting to discuss the draft to ensure accuracy and acceptance of the report. Some participants will indicate their comments need additional context, or have been 'misunderstood'; then clarifications can be made.

Incidentally, in another session of the same consultation process in another state with different participants, individual acknowledgment of input was requested by all concerned. The learning outcome for me was a reminder to listen, observe and adapt to the context, environment and timing of *every* participatory process, that is, *conscious contextuality*. Awareness and inclusion of local situation processes may result in *human-centred solutions*, suggestions for and commitment to new developments from the people involved.

It's lovely work, but qualitative research still has to pay the bills ...

When I started my business, a consultant friend warned that government clients always expect more than is contracted. I thought this was exaggerated, but it is proven true in my experience.

My understanding of this phenomenon is that, as receivers of a regular wage, as long as they have a working relationship with you, government staff unconsciously work on an assumption that as a consultant you are there for their project alone. I have, however, worked with the rare senior public servant who recognizes the realities of operating in a commercial market, who will adapt a contract's details to authorize and pay for extra work as well as facilitate timely payment. Most do not have this understanding. Many government employees have no experience or understanding of commercial realities, including the concept that the only thing a consultant has to sell is time and expertise, in a time-limited environment with no paid sick leave or holidays, and no guarantee of regular paid work.

I now have strategies to secure payment for what I do:

- Include in every contract the daily or hourly costs for extra work outside the scope of the original project's cost.
- Negotiate to change standard government contract clauses about invoicing from thirty-day payment to 'on receipt of invoice'. The 'thirty days' is often interpreted internally to start from when the approved invoice arrives in the accounts section, even if it has taken weeks for approval

with the authorized signatures, and that is months after the work is accepted as satisfactory.[7]

Qualitative research – a challenging career

There is no doubt an advanced degree or a PhD helps convince clients that their projects are in responsible hands, but it is no automatic magnet attracting paid work. The need for constant self-marketing is demanding and is opposed to the inclinations of introverts who may feel that research is a quiet way to earn a living.

In this postmodern deconstructed world of multiple careers, there is no permanent job security. Qualitative research skills are useful life skills that, once learned, are always a part of experience, enriching our knowledge and competencies with practice.

We can explore the territory (scoping). We can inquire into complex situations that may provide income-generating opportunities. We can consult with likely game players and look for bottom-up opportunities to strengthen our communities. We can tell the story of the society we live in with our ability to stand aside and make meaning out of it all (meta-analysis). Most importantly, we can apply our creative imagination to problem solving that can (in some cases) improve the quality of life for our nation and our community, and thus ourselves.

> *Problems cannot be solved at the same level of awareness that created them.* *(Einstein, quoted as a headline by Salter, 2000, p. 238)*

Qualitative research skills provide the capacity to tell the stories of our communities, further enhancing our understanding of why we experience the world as we do. Meta-analysis requires that we stand aside and reflect upon the stories. With this understanding, we have more capacity to work creatively with the change that is all around us.

I am curious to see what comes next in my career, in my creative life, in my community and my country. I am committed to the process of inquiry to uncover the stories of why we, in our various communities, experience the world as we do: *conscious contextuality*. It is the messiness of qualitative research that fleshes out the bones, gives shape and meaning to statistics and more fully informs government about public policy, that can strengthen and enhance communities. I guess I will stay here for a while, playing in the mud. It is even more fun when other researchers, community members, interest groups, NGOs and government people come to play too; together we reshape sustainable futures, experiencing *sacred encounters*. Through qualitative research we can discover the stories within people, from which we uncover and develop their own *human-centred solutions*.

[1] Thich Nhat Hahn, a Vietnamese Buddhist monk, is quoted in a management journal which condenses 'good advice about leading and inspiring people' *(Bits and Pieces*, R(2), 11).
[2] I refer to grounded feminist theory that puts feminist social justice into action, as practised by Gunew and Yeatman (1993), hooks (1984), Peavey (1994), Reinharz (1992) and many other practitioners with pragmatic social justice in mind.
[3] I looked for good practice through collaborative inquiry with twelve women, and through analysis of management practices in Australia and internationally (e.g. Roddick, 1991; Semler, 1993).

[4] The first career was a teacher over 25 years (from kindergarten to Year 12, primary school, adult learning and training, university); the second was a mother; the third was community development; the fourth was workplace trainer/learning consultant. Then in my fifth decade I evolved into a research consultant.

[5] As Stella Cornelius described her work in my PhD thesis. Now in her late 70s, she continues to be a strong activist for peace through the Conflict Resolution network. In December 2000, she arranged to send a team of mediators to Burma.

[6] The process for a health professional education promotion (started 6 months after the family project) included air fares for a number of face-to-face meetings as well as a reduction in the number of experts needed for text approval.

[7] As I did the last edit on this chapter I received a phone call from a public servant apologizing for the delayed payment of two invoices due to the department changing its payment system from one programme to another. From acceptance of report and delivery of invoice to receipt of payment totalled 13 weeks past due in this instance. By the way, no-one is at fault, '. . . that's just the way it is'.

References

Gunew, S. and Yeatman, A. (eds) (1993) *Feminism and the Politics of Difference.* Sydney: Allen and Unwin.

hooks, b. (1984) *Feminist Theory: From Margin to Center.* Boston: South East End Press.

Kaufman Hall, V. (1996) *Women Transforming the Workplace – Collaborative Inquiry Into Integrity in Action.* PhD thesis, University of Western Sydney, Hawkesbury, Australia.

Kaufman Hall, V. (1998) *Nursing Mothers' Association of Australia, National Breastfeeding Education/Promotion – Family Project – Evaluation and Final Report* (in consultation with NMAA Board, staff and Project Officers, Statistics – Vicki Grieve) for Commonwealth Department of Health, Canberra, Australia.

National Inquiry Into the Separation of Aboriginal and Torres Strait Islander Children From Their Families (1997) *Bringing Them Home.* Sydney: Human Rights and Equal Opportunity Commission, Commonwealth of Australia.

Oxford Dictionary of Quotations (1985), 3rd edn, p. 573. London: Guild Publishing.

Peavey, F. (1994) *By Life's Grace – Musings on the Essence of Social Change.* Philadelphia: New Society Publishers.

Pusey, M. (1991) *Economic Rationalism in Canberra: A Nation-Building State Changes Its Mind.* Sydney: Cambridge University Press.

Reason, P. (ed.) (1994) *Collaborative Inquiry.* Centre for the Study of Organizational Change and Development, University of Bath, Bath, UK.

Reinharz, S. (1992) *Feminist Methods in Social Research.* Oxford: Oxford University Press.

Roddick, A. (1991) *Body and Soul.* London: Edbury.

Salter, C. (2000) We're trying to change world history. In *Fast Company*, vol. 40, pp. 230–238.

Semler, R. (1993) *Maverick! The Success Story Behind the World's Most Unusual Workplace.* London: Century.

Thich Nhat Hahn (1991) *Peace is Every Step.* New York: Bantam.

Wilson, R. (2000) *A Big Ask – Interviews With Interviewers.* Amsterdam: New Holland.

Legislation

Section 165-55 of A New Tax System (Goods and Services Tax) Act 1999 (No. 55) (Cwlth); *http://scaleplus.law.gov.au*

10

Learning through supervising

David Smith

I have always been strongly committed to the notion that experience can be a powerful teacher. We spend our lives experiencing, and this is just as true in the role of supervisor as for any other role we play. I have also strongly asserted the caveat that we do not necessarily optimize our learning from our experience. The only way this occurs, I believe, is in finding strategies, either individually or, preferably, with others, to reflect: to find time and space to detach from the experience and reconsider it through recreating it, reframing it, looking at it from different points of view, being challenged about our assumptions and perceptions related to the experience and considering different alternatives and possibilities. There are many strategies for reflection to turn experience into learning.

One very powerful strategy for reflection and learning is writing about the experience. Thus, the request to write this chapter provides a very special opportunity for me to reflect on my learning as a supervisor over some sixteen years of working with undergraduate and postgraduate researchers. Because of the nature of the task, my chapter will be personal, and probably different from the usual academic genre. I begin by making some comments on the nature and purpose of the supervision experience and its potential for learning. I then discuss several specific examples of my learning that have been particularly important and powerful.

On the nature of supervision

In my experience, each research supervision and the biographic and institutional circumstances in which it is embedded are unique. Each has its own path, its own journey, its own periods of highs and lows, its own times of challenge, of confrontation and celebration. One of the research candidates I supervised once wrote about her journey in the words of a well-known song, 'one day a diamond, next day a stone'. Somehow, this seems to capture at least some aspects of the research journey.

The major purpose of any research supervision is, from my point of view, apart from assisting someone to gain a qualification and credential, to assist a future academic colleague to develop the skills, awarenesses, commitments and understandings to become a successful researcher and an effective worker within the context of the university and the international life of an academic. There are, of course, different models and metaphors possible to describe the supervisory process. Some are fairly didactic, such as the model of the neophyte researcher sitting at the feet of the expert. But supervision can be considered much more as a mentoring role in which the supervisor acts as a more experienced colleague to assist the research candidate to acquire the necessary skills and understandings to be a successful academic, both within the confines of the institution and, just as importantly, in the wider contexts of national and international meetings and conferences and in decisions relating to an academic career.

Thus supervision by its very nature is educational – it is a purposeful teaching and learning experience. Usually this experience is considered mainly from the point of view of the people being supervised and their learning, not only about the skills and understandings of becoming a researcher, but often also about becoming an effective future supervisor. However, as in any teaching/learning experience, supervision also provides powerful potential for the supervisor's learning. As in all learning situations there is the opportunity for the supervisor to learn about a variety of things; what is learned will depend to some extent on the context of the supervision and the subjectivities of the individuals involved.

Probably the most obvious learning potential for the supervisor lies in the opportunity, through the supervision, to learn even more about the subject of the research. I have always felt that to be a supervisor is a special privilege, partly because of the opportunity it presents to be kept in contact with the very latest research and writing in the subject area being supervised. In saying this, of course, I can imagine some of the 'shock, horror' reactions of some university academics, who may support the stereotype myth that a supervisor is selected on the basis of being one of the most knowledgeable people in the field of the proposed research. I call this a myth, because in my experience as a university supervisor there has not been one thesis for which I would call myself 'expert'. Although I may have been knowledgeable about some aspect of either the substantive area or the methodology being employed in some of the theses I have supervised, there were always aspects of the research and/or research context about which I knew very little. In addition, there have been a number of theses I have had to supervise for which, at the commencement of the candidature, I had little knowledge about the area at all. All academics, if they are honest, know that for a variety of reasons we are asked to supervise in areas in which we are not 'expert'. As an ex-Associate Dean for Postgraduate Studies and also for Research, I appreciate the problematic nature of such supervisions. I would also argue that, in my experience at least, these challenges often occur, and, further, they often present opportunities for the most powerful learning. Apart from these types of candidature, however, even if a candidate approaches you as a supervisor because of your reputation as a researcher and writer in a particular area, that does not necessarily mean that you have access to, or continue to have access to, the very latest knowledge that can inform the candidate's work. It is likely that a research candidate will, because of the singular focus on a reasonably defined area, find material that you as supervisor are not necessarily familiar with. This is part of the privilege of being a supervisor, and a powerful opportunity for co-learning.

A second potential area for learning lies in the area of human interaction and communication. Fundamentally, for me, supervision is about relationships and communication. Those relationships are based, I would assert, in a mutuality of respect and trust and a commitment to the completion of the research by both parties, as well as an interest in the topics/questions being investigated. If either the candidate or the supervisor does not contribute to this mutual relationship, then it is difficult for the supervisory process and for the research candidature to be completed. Thus a supervisor learns a lot about the people supervised: their nature and characteristics, and the manner in which they respond to a wide variety of situations and challenges. In turn, such learning enhances understanding of humans, their motivations, behaviour and interactions.

Thirdly, however, and most importantly, any supervision experience provides a powerful opportunity for supervisors to learn about themselves. Because supervision, like any form of teaching, may be characterized as a fairly intense interactive relationship, as a supervisor you are constantly being provided with feedback about your ideas and yourself. In addition, because supervision is characterized by a high level of complex oral interaction you have powerful opportunities to learn about your skills in communication, particularly skills related to listening with understanding and empathy and to clarity in explanation of often highly abstract ideas. The opportunity for such learning is further enhanced if the candidate with whom you are working comes from a language and/or cultural background other than your own.

Choosing to provide specific opportunities to reflect together on the experience and process of the supervision and making it work more effectively for candidate and supervisor, I know, is a further means to enhance the potential for learning, and I now build this activity into every supervision experience. Sometimes it occurs on a one-to-one basis. It has also been part of the activities of a research support group that I and a number of my research candidates established and fostered. The group served a number of purposes. It acted principally as a support group for all members, a place where the 'elders', who were further along in their journeys, could share stories of the 'rituals' of the institutional context, such as the process of the development of thesis proposals, the thesis committee experience, and dealing with the bureaucracy of the university. The group was also an important venue for sharing problems and challenges and celebrating successes, such as successful thesis committees, the finishing of draft chapters and then of the thesis, submission of the thesis and successful examination and graduation; often, it seems, there does not appear to be celebration of important milestones along the research journey. Equally important, group meetings provided a forum for the sharing of ideas related to the substance of topics or to aspects of methodology, discussion of drafts of conference papers, proposals and chapters. Often meetings were based on papers recently published that related to aspects of one person's work but which provided further opportunities for learning for both candidates and the supervisor.

The importance of research candidature experience

I believe that the manner in which you approach supervision, as well as its potential for your own learning, have a great deal to do with your own experience as a research candidate. While I know of no published work related to the relationship between supervisors' beliefs and behaviour and their previous experience as a supervisee, I can certainly point to numerous tension points and anecdotes of research candidatures that are often illuminated by a comment from a supervisor, such as, 'well, I had to do that', or 'well, that was the way I was treated'. It seems that sometimes those who come after us have to endure our experiences even when they are often no longer relevant. This also highlights the fact that being a supervisor also provides an opportunity to learn about another facet of the workplace, that is, one's colleagues.

Arguably, then, if one's experience of being supervised is an important factor, I should tell you of something of my own experience and how that has acted as a catalyst in my learning. My doctorate was completed part-time during the early 1980s, while I was a full-time academic. It was one of the first non-quantitative doctoral studies to be completed in the department, and thus had all the imaginable difficulties and advantages of 'trail blazing' in a reasonably traditional university environment. Because I was a staff member, the university required that I be supervised by one of the three professors. My supervisor was an experienced teacher and educational researcher with an excellent Australian and international reputation. He had highly developed skills as a writer and editor. There is no doubt that these were invaluable for me, and that many of the skills, if any, that I possess in academic writing I would attribute to him and his supervision of my work.

At the same time, however, my supervisor was in the same position that I have described above for myself and others as supervisors; that is, he knew very little about the substantive area of my research dealing with teacher decision-making. Despite this, what was successful in my supervisory process was the relationship that we had with one another. I respected him as an academic, both in his own right and as someone who knew the university context in which I was working as a research candidate, with its culture, procedures and regulations. I trusted him to be able to navigate me through to a successful conclusion. For my part, I perceived that my supervisor respected me as a person, and the quality of my work. While he did not necessarily always agree with my ideas, and provided constant critical judgment of my writing, he accepted my input when I was able to provide reasonable defences for what I thought and wrote, and he respected my scholarship. Often we would have strong disagreements, even arguments, about some aspects of my work. In many ways, however, I now believe that it was because of this context that I was forced to develop strong confidence concerning the quality and validity of my own work. Because I knew that my supervisor was not 'the expert' in my field, I had to make sure that I really understood what I was doing to ensure the quality of my research and writing.

I also learned at that time about the risk involved in presenting particularly one's written ideas to another reader, a lesson that, I think, has been important in how I approach my supervision now. While I accept that critique is a fundamental principle of academic work and publication, it is somewhat easier to endure after some successful experience. I still well remember working on a chapter draft until I believed it was the best possible, then with trepidation submitting it to my supervisor and waiting anxiously for the appointment after he had read it. Those experiences and their attendant feelings are important to me now in working with others. I believe that those memories help me to be empathetic and understanding of others' anxieties when I am the reader of their work. I know that positive and constructive critique will facilitate effective completion of their candidature.

While it was my supervisor who made the final decision regarding the submission of my thesis for examination, in many ways the responsibility for ensuring the accuracy of my methodology and the quality of the research, the data and its investigation was my own. When my thesis was submitted, I had to be confident that it would successfully pass the scrutiny of its international examiners. Even though I was confident of the quality of my work and its scholarship and, now as a supervisor, I understand the sometimes anxious period between when a thesis is sent out for examination and the examiners' reports are received, I believe that it was not until my international examiners had passed a more than satisfactory judgment on my thesis that my supervisor really understood the quality of my work.

I believe that my experience of being supervised taught me a number of important things that are significant in my work as a supervisor. First, I came to understand that effective supervision derives from a successful relationship based on mutual trust and respect, which provides the basis of authentic communication. I am not necessarily saying that this ideal was always realized, but it is substantiated as much in its absence as in its presence. Further, I believe that power and the manner in which it is negotiated (or not negotiated) is a central aspect of all relationships. This is also true of the supervisory relationship. Different models for supervision reflect alternatives for dealing with this issue of power. In the 'expert' model, power is usually asymmetrically distributed. Alternatively, in a model of co-learning power is more dynamic and shifts from one to the other according to the context and purposes. I experienced examples of both these approaches at different points during my candidature, and my feelings and reactions to them, which are still vivid, inform my work as a supervisor. I did not enjoy someone holding power over me and my work, especially when it was positional power and not power derived from a thorough understanding of the subject matter in question. Thus, while I would argue that there are times in most candidatures (e.g. in matters related to procedures, protocols and practices of research candidature in a specific university; at times of legitimate and necessary confrontation relating to unsatisfactory commitment or progress) where as supervisor I need to take responsibility and act as the 'expert', most of the time I aspire to negotiating power in interactions, discussions and decisions, and I deliberately work towards an increasing empowerment of candidates in matters related to their work.

Second, I learned that because supervising is about relationship, knowing everything about a topic is not the most important ingredient of a successful research supervision. It certainly helps to know something about the research candidate's topic; however, I would argue that what is even more important is whether an effective professional relationship can be established between the supervisor and the candidate. Like all relationships, it evolves successfully only if people are committed to it and take the time to work together to make it happen.

Third, I also learned that supervisions can be successful and do not necessarily have to be traumatic, impossibly challenging or attenuated. Because of my experience of relatively smooth success, I approach every candidature as supervisor with the expectation that it will be successful. As part of this attitude, it is my strong belief that while successful research candidates require a modicum of intelligence and ability, it is not high intelligence that is the most important factor in a successful research candidature. Of much more importance is a disciplined and tenacious, conscientious commitment to work, and an ability to sustain it over an extended period. Thus I begin all supervision with a strong expectation and conviction that it will be successful, and I communicate this explicitly to the candidate both at the beginning of the process and at critical times when things get difficult along the journey.

The fourth and, I consider, most important learning from my experience of being supervised, which has had the most impact on my role as supervisor, was confidence in my own judgment. This confidence stemmed, I believe, at least partly from the experience of having to be largely responsible for judgments about the quality of my research and writing and its readiness for international peer scrutiny. My judgments were vindicated by the affirmation of those examiners. What this means is that, after carefully examining the work of candidates, I trust the judgments that I make and am prepared to stand by them, even when the area of the thesis is not one in which I would claim expert knowledge. This original confidence has been reinforced on at least two occasions when other colleagues, after reading candidates' final drafts, have suggested what amounted to major revisions, which would have extended the candidature unreasonably. The first of these examples was with my very first doctoral supervision, so I certainly did not have much experience of research supervision at that point. In addition, the candidate happened to be a colleague in my department, and the revisions were suggested by a professor and head of department. Thus the stakes were fairly high. After what I believed to be an effective supervisory process, and after careful reading of the final draft to be submitted, I believed that it was ready for examination by international peers. My decision was proved to be correct, and thus this experience provided further confidence for me in the accuracy of my judgment in the supervisory process.

In summary, I am convinced that supervisory style, particularly in relation to issues of power and control, is often strongly influenced by the supervisor's previous experience of being supervised. This refers not only to the model of supervision employed, but also, and interrelated with it, to the manner in which power is negotiated (or not) in the supervisory relationship, and the predisposition the supervisor has to the potential for learning from the supervisory experience. If your previous experience as a supervisee was successful and relatively unproblematic, then you are likely to have positive predispositions towards the candidature and its outcome, towards your relationship with the candidate, and towards your own learning. Alternatively, it seems possible that if your experience was more negative, problematic and attenuated, this may translate into a less positive predisposition. The predisposition of the supervisor can be particularly important at certain critical points in a candidature.

Learning in the spiral of supervision

Initially, a successful relationship is often based upon the supervisor being willing to take a leadership role and communicate confidence about the successful completion of the research and thesis – even if the signs are not immediately evident; for me, the tension is between building confidence in the candidate to complete the project and at the same time being realistic about the difficulties of doing so as the confidence-building continues. In these early phases in particular the role of the supervisor is very much the experienced other, the mentor, standing alongside and possibly even more leading the neophyte through the labyrinth of protocol, rules, regulations and procedures to establish the research project, develop the proposal through the stages of acceptance and get it to a point of viable beginning.

Arguably, as already indicated, the key element of a successful relationship, especially at this stage, is effective communication. Particularly important are aspects of active listening and dealing with feelings of anxiety, frustration, anger, and possibly loss of confidence and self esteem. In addition, it is not only negotiating meaning through honest and direct assertive communication that is important, but also establishing the parameters and 'rules' for setting session agendas, prioritizing issues and providing possibilities for reflecting.

In this early phase the self-confidence of the supervisor, the belief in the potential to bring the supervision to a successful conclusion, and the clear communication of these attitudes to the candidate are important. This explicit confidence and its communication to the candidate are, I would argue, important in helping to develop and sustain the confidence of the candidate in successfully completing the task. This confidence of the candidate is an important factor in the continued long-term commitment to completing the research and thesis successfully. Wavering confidence threatens commitment because of a decline in belief in the successful completion of the project.

The supervisory relationship is dynamic; it changes as the candidate becomes more confident and experienced in undertaking the research and managing the project and its report. Indeed, the supervisory relationship can be seen as two 'V's, with one inverse to the other. The first represents the candidate, who gradually increases over the time of the relationship in confidence and responsibility for the work. The inverse is the role of the supervisor, who gradually assumes less direct responsibility for the management of the project.

In my experience, the most typical learning context relating to supervision is one in which the supervisor and candidate come together to discuss an issue, a problem or, particularly in the later stages, a draft of writing by the candidate. Whatever the issue/problem/product, like any learning situation, there are elements of risk and ownership to be negotiated. While often these may be seen to belong to the candidate (in that it is the candidate's problem or writing that is being discussed), it is also the opinions, ideas and comments/reactions of the supervisor that are being risked regarding the reactions of the candidate. As in any teaching relationship, the pupil and the teacher are equally potentially confronted by themselves, their interactions and their relationship. Again, it depends on the specific approach to supervision that is being employed. For me, the interactions are characterized by a negotiation of meaning in which each participant dynamically adopts shifting positions of 'expert' through to 'novice', depending on what is being addressed at any particular moment. Sometimes the supervisor is expert and the candidate is novice, sometimes the reverse. Such negotiation, if it is to occur effectively, demands large amounts of time. Increasingly, the demand to teach more students with less staff means that such time is often not possible, and consequently as a supervisor you are pushed into adopting a more didactic supervisory approach.

Research supervision provides an exciting and powerful stimulus for learning by both the candidate and the supervisor. The candidate learns not only advanced skills in research, project management, reporting and writing, but also important insights into the supervisory process through the modelling of the supervisor. In addition, candidates are confronted by themselves, with important potentials for knowing, being and becoming who they are. Similarly, supervisors not only add to their experience of the challenges of supervision as an intense sequence of human relationships and interactions and how to manage it all in a university context; they, too, are presented with important opportunities for learning about themselves and for their own knowing, being and becoming. The degree to which such learning occurs, however, arguably depends on the predispositions of the supervisor towards the nature and practice of research supervision.

11

Sparks fly: when life, work and research collide

Martin Mulligan

Above my desk at work these days is a black-and-white photograph of two alert babies staring inquisitively at the camera. When I look at the photo and then close my eyes their faces become animated; they fill with colour and are softened by engaging smiles. Those two faces are never far from my thoughts now because they belong to my passionate and volatile son, Roshan Nemaluk Mulligan, and his calm and curious twin sister, Indu Maeve Mulligan. They are faces that became imprinted on my mind when Indu stared deeply into my soul and Roshan nestled comfortably into the crook of my arm on the day they were born in December 1998.

I was on study leave from my job as a university lecturer when the twins arrived, and part of my study became an intensive refresher course in parenting skills (my other son was already 21). It was experiential learning with no opportunity to go home after the classes. Sharply conflicting advice from family and friends only confused the matter. Our lives had been thrown into thrilling but unnerving chaos. Two months later I returned to my 'normal' work routine, but now I had both a compelling reason and strong desire to be very selective in my work priorities. It was the only way I could begin to identify some patterns in the chaos that had engulfed me.

I found I had much in common with Ken, a PhD student I was supervising. He had also become a father again after a long interregnum. 'Wow, you forget how demanding this is, don't you?' he said when we met (and he only had one baby to deal with!). 'But there's no way I would want to send her back', he continued. 'I feel incredibly close to her. Having her has made me think a lot about what I value in life.' We agreed that when this heavy responsibility is dropped into your arms you have to find a way to carry it, because the sack contains nuggets of gold as well as potatoes.

Ken has been using ideas from chaos and complexity science (Waldrop, 1994) in his work on creativity within organizations. Waldrop explains that theories of chaos and complexity suggest that stability is death, and chaos is the source of creativity. Chaos adds complexity, and patterns form at the 'edge of chaos'. Things cycle between apparent order and chaos. That sounds like a fair description of parenthood, we agreed. Let's hope that the transitory patterns last for a while, I offered. Only if they are complex and adaptive, Ken responded, referring again to the theory.

In our Western culture we learn to fear chaos. Order and predictability are treasured; we even have traditions of trying to emulate machines in the way we organize our lives (mechanistic thinking). But try as we might to maintain control, disorder always finds a way of poking its nose in to set off some chaotic events that can amplify through our well-ordered systems. We might, for example, design the perfect research project, only to find we are inexorably dragged in a different direction. We can learn to 'go with the flow' and look for opportunities in the disturbances. But we have to overcome cultural prejudices in order to befriend chaos and discover its creative power. Even then, we can't help worrying when things seem 'out of control'.

I'm one of those people who periodically makes lists of 'Things To Do' when I'm at my office desk. (I also tend to make mental lists about what I want to achieve outside work.) The good thing about such lists is that you can get great satisfaction out of scratching off a completed task, especially if it has stubbornly announced itself on list after list. Lists can also be good for browsing and thinking about priorities before getting lost in a particular task. The down side is that you are even more aware of the number of tasks jostling for your attention. You can get stressed out just thinking about where to begin and, just as your mental anguish reaches a peak, new tasks and possibilities thud onto your desk or lob into your life. Since becoming a father again, my lists have actually become shorter. That's because an unlisted item – how to be a decent father – magically forces other items off the page. Parenthood imposes itself on all my agendas because it is an imperative rather than a priority. As Ken said, it makes you think more deeply about what's important. But surely there are easier ways of finding focus?

Of course there are, but it's not just a matter of focus. It's more a matter of tapping into some kind of life force, for want of a better term. Campaigning for social justice was a life force for me for many years; deep immersion in social and political change movements. Success was limited and often temporary; my motivation waned and my focus became fractured. A new job in the innovative School of Social Ecology at the University of Western Sydney, Hawkesbury, offered new opportunities and new incentives, but again the frustrations began to accumulate. What seems different about parenthood as a life force is that it extends your sense of self, but not too far. As I wrote in a poem recently (see end of chapter), the thrilling but terrifying thought that confronts me now is that 'I am three and three is me'. My direct stake in the future has suddenly been expanded and extended, way beyond my own expected lifespan. Having achieved a 'mature' age I can be a more conscious parent this time around; more fully aware of what I can bring to the job (even if the energy levels aren't what they once were!). That's what is helping me to re-evaluate what I am doing in my work as a teacher and in my research (see later). That's the way a life force, whatever it might be, can change the questions about priorities. I am still faced with a multitude of choices, but I feel that my extended sense of self will help me make choices that are ethically sound. And working out how to make ethical choices seems to be a fundamental requirement of our time.

Writer and psychotherapist Michael Ventura (1995) has suggested that we have entered 'the age of interruption', when we are constantly bombarded by information and disturbances from a wide range of sources: telephone, television, radio, Internet, email, and face-to-face conversations. We put recording machines on our phones and find we have messages that demand an instant response. Some of us have a 'call waiting' facility, and try to have more than one telephone conversation at once (a pet hate of mine). It is often difficult to have a 'live' conversation that isn't interrupted by telephone calls or other people barging in. Our attention is fractured or, at best, thinly spread. So-called time saving devices, from motorcars to email, simply mean that we try to fit more into the time available. As Ventura wrote, we fill our lives with a 'busyness' that defies contemplation and serious pursuit of the particular. 'Background noise' has been foregrounded, and it is difficult to decide what is important. Of course, new technologies also enable us to join multiple discourses that can bring us into contact with many interesting ideas in a short space of time. We can join special interest conversations that might even have a global reach. However, more than ever we have to make choices about the discourses we will join, and our capacity to choose well is more an assessment of personal values than a technical skill. More than ever, our use of time is a matter of value judgments.

In a book on ethics in an era of globalization, Peter Singer (1995) wrote that, more than ever, we are obliged to think carefully about the likely consequences of our actions for other people and other living things (both near and far). Abstract principles for guiding ethical behaviour are of little assistance when we live in a chaotic, complex and increasingly interdependent world. What we do in one situation might differ from what we decide is ethical behaviour in different circumstances. According to Singer, we need an applied form of ethics in which we actively contemplate the likely consequences of what we plan to do.

For me, the task is made easier by having a broader sense of self. My aim is to make choices that enhance life for Indu and Roshan so that they might also learn to love and respect life. My concern is not limited to the twins – my teaching and research is aimed at a much broader audience – but it is a useful test to consider the consequences of what I do for those whose lives are most closely entwined with mine. Perhaps the discredited 'trickle-down effect' (i.e., the notion that we will all eventually benefit if the 'economy' is strong) might be replaced by the 'ripple-out effect' of ethical decision-making. You don't have to be a parent of infant children to have an outward-oriented sense of self, and I'm not smugly suggesting that parenthood is the answer (it can also be a disaster). I'm just trying to illustrate how an embodied sense of responsibility for other, real people can help us to make ethical, life-enhancing decisions regarding our own life and work. Let me illustrate this with an example of my recent thought processes.

At the time of writing this chapter, my main research project involved writing a book about 'the emergence of ecological understandings in Australia' with friend and colleague Stuart Hill. For this book we took a broad view of what constitutes ecological understandings, seeing their emergence in fields ranging from biological sciences to landscape art and the Aboriginal land rights movement. To make the book more accessible, we decided to focus on the life and work of selected 'key people' who have made innovative contributions in a range of fields. In conducting research for the book, which included lengthy interviews with some of the key people, I had to develop a literacy in some fields that were previously outside my domain (e.g. landscape art). I was challenged to think about contributions I might be able to make towards the promotion of ecological understandings (leading to significant changes to subjects I teach). And I was prompted to think about my own identity; for example, what does it mean to associate myself with the nature conservation movement and hope to be part of its future? Increasingly, I am thinking about what I might be able to share from all of this with the twins as they grow into greater consciousness. Interviewing pioneer conservationists made me understand better why bushwalking and camping have been important to me. I have new ways of appreciating artists and writers. I dream of taking the twins to revisit Aboriginal communities in the Northern Territory where the modern Aboriginal land rights movement started in the 1960s, so that they might get some sense of how these people see the land. I will have stories to share with the twins about land and identity in Australia; stories that were not available to me as a child. Given that my wife is Sri Lankan, the twins will grow up with many interesting questions and challenges about their identity.

Another example. Over a number of years I have been developing a subject called 'Wilderness Values and Landscape Conservation'. We critically examine cultural concepts embedded in words like 'wilderness' and 'landscape', and discuss the need to overcome nature/culture dualisms. I take some of the students on walking trips into wilderness areas and get all of them to explore a 'sense of place' in a location near where they live. We discuss ideas around bioregionalism and 'reading storied landscapes'. In my teaching and recent writing I have been arguing the importance of sensuous experiences of wildness (not wilderness) for developing respect for the non-human world. I had many sensuous experiences of nature growing up on the edge of Sydney, and I want to ensure that the twins have some similar experiences. However, my Sri Lankan wife and her hyper-cautious family worry about the dangers I might expose them to. Ideas that I advocate in my teaching and research have to be the subject of negotiation in my own life. I am faced with making ethical choices around my hopes and responsibilities – a rigorous test of what I advocate.

One of the problems we face is that, historically, we have segmentary ways of thinking. Our culture is dominated by 'rational' modes of thought that owe much to the forms of logic articulated by Plato and Aristotle. Some scholars (see McKeon, 1987) have said that Aristotle's legacy, in particular, has been severely distorted; Aristotle himself pointed out that the rules of 'formal logic' (i.e. rationalism) are useful for solving only particular kinds of problems. In other circumstances Aristotle favoured the art of rhetorical discourse, in which participants would take turns to construct explanatory arguments that would be assessed for their aesthetics as well as their explanatory power. Participants in such an exercise are encouraged to enjoy exploring the nuances of language. In being pushed aside by rationalism, the word 'rhetoric' has been turned into an insult, and we have lost the art of this kind of discourse. Some feminist scholars (e.g. Lloyd, 1984; Belenky *et al.*, 1986) have argued that the dominance of rationalism is related to the hegemony of patriarchal ideas in our culture. Belenky *et al.* argue that we need to rehabilitate 'women's ways of knowing', including the skilful use of intuition.

In making applied ethical decisions we frequently draw from conscious and unconscious experience to do what we 'feel' will be right for ourselves and other people (i.e., we use intuition). We have to use non-linear (i.e. non-rational) modes of thought to contemplate the ripple-out (and ripple-back) impacts of our actions. Intuitively and pragmatically, we know that we live in a chaotic world, in which rational modes of thought have only limited value, yet we persist with the limited conceptual tools that are made available to us.

We try to impose order on a chaotic world by creating conceptual compartments. We seek to isolate particular 'problems' or sets of problems, to be analysed by people with 'technical skill' in the field in which the problems are thought to have arisen. We segregate one profession from another, and the professional from the private. Much of this compartmentalization is useful for making some sense of overwhelming complexity and for communicating our limited experiences and understandings with others. But we can run into problems when we mistake our conceptual ordering of the world for reality. People engaged in a sustained research project, for example, commonly find that they have to pursue their 'problem' across the boundaries of academic disciplines and professional expertise. And what might start as a professional concern will often travel home with the researcher. A recently completed PhD project that I supervised began as an exploration of teaching practices in the classroom and became a largely autobiographical exploration of ideas and influences that help us make sense of our relationships with other people, the contexts including that of the classroom (Byrne-Armstrong, 1999). If we are engaged in social research, it is difficult to imagine how we could maintain a segregation of the personal and professional. Dialogues we have with other people, including authors we read, frequently reflect back on us personally. Conversely, significant events in our personal lives can change the way we think about our professional activities. That has certainly been my experience in relearning how to be a parent: a task that draws heavily on intuition.

Marilyn Waring (1996) and others have pointed out that the separation of 'life' and 'work' involves some extraordinary classifications and erasures. Isn't the work that women (mostly) do in the home just as important for society as the work people do in paid employment? Yet it is made less valuable by being excluded from the moneyed economy, and frequently hidden from sight. Similarly, the vast amount of volunteer work that people do in community organizations, family businesses and so on is frequently undervalued and hidden. We fail to acknowledge the skill and wisdom of those who have become highly skilled in unpaid work. Their voices are rarely heard. Home-making skills and personal research projects are often dismissed as 'hobbies'.

Some of us are lucky enough to be paid for doing what we (largely) enjoy doing. We may even be encouraged to pursue our personal research interests at work. For many more, however, paid work is tedious and unfulfilling, related only to the need for an income. In this case research interests are more likely to be associated with 'life interests' that must be pursued outside 'work time'. I often advise people wanting to undertake research degrees at university to choose topics that can blur the boundaries between 'life' and 'work'; that can undermine the tyranny of this segregation. As many readers will know, a sustained research project can be a long, hard slog, and the desire to complete the project must be strong enough to withstand days of withering confusion and doubt, and times when progress is highly elusive. Projects that can enhance both work and life experiences have the best chance of continually stimulating the creative juices.

A starting point may be nagging questions that won't go away, or feelings of discomfort and self-doubt that are demanding attention. Then there's the 'I've got a book in me' syndrome, where the researcher sets out to test the quality of ideas that might eventually materialize in book form. Others may simply be attracted by the challenge of sustained scholarship, and, of course, research qualifications may be a way of opening up new career opportunities. The starting points are diverse, but all researchers need a strong motivation to reach some kind of completion. Perhaps the strongest motivations are those that can be easily related back to core values. Another PhD student I am supervising was recently thrown into deep dismay when her research on community attitudes to marine life in intertidal coastal zones was sharply attacked by two marine biologists with whom she was working. However, she was able to find a way out of this crisis by returning to her strong motivation for reducing damaging human impacts on intertidal ecosystems. In an earlier project, she had written passionately and personally about her deep love of the sea and the coast (Hemery, 1995).

We can consciously blur the boundaries between life, work and research when we look for overlapping interests, projects and discourses. We can learn to love the creative chaos that this involves. But we will also experience frustration and despair when we are torn apart by competing priorities or overcome by a sense of failure. We might reconceive life and work as artificially constructed conceptual categories, but we all know that they often seem to collide, sometimes with terrifying force. These different segments of our lives sometimes collide with such force that sparks fly, leading to heated arguments or smouldering tensions. In the chaotic interactions of conflict we may discover the spark of a new idea or we may even find that our lives re-emerge in a new form, like a Phoenix rising from the ashes.

As mentioned, I have found that fatherhood has turned some priorities into imperatives, thus hardening the boundaries. This means that the collisions of life and work are likely to have even more impact; sending more sparks flying. It certainly isn't easy to combine fatherhood with full-time paid employment and a strong desire to pursue research projects (that can't be solely confined to work). In my worse moments, fuelled no doubt by chronic sleep deprivation, I have terrible visions of segments of my life being like several fast-moving trains converging on the same intersection from different directions. A fearsome and destructive collision seems inevitable. But more often, I think in terms of the metaphor captured by the wonderful phrase 'we make our path by walking'.[1] Immersed in a challenging landscape, I have to draw on all my experience to blaze a trail ahead. Confusion and despair disorient me. Some other people want to push me off the path I have created. But when I get overheated, I look around to remind myself that my family is travelling with me. We will not always agree about which way we should head. Sometimes we will follow different paths, at least for a while. But we will also make time to sit down, build a little fire, boil a billy, and talk about our journey and the landscapes we are traversing. The experience is enriched in the sharing.

My advice to others who would willingly add research work to already crowded lives? Expect the unexpected and rely on your core values to make applied ethical judgments about the best path to follow. Work on your capacity to think broadly and flexibly. And, above all, if the research you are doing fails to bring you enjoyment and/or satisfaction, then think again. As the French like to say 'Life is too short . . . '.

Linking thoughts

I'm sitting in the Linking Cave[2]
as swirling winds and drifting rain
are drifting out of focus.
And down below my feet I see
a dusty pathway falling steeply
then more gently undulating
into a sea of mist.

That path, I know, leads back to Sydney
down through space and time,
back to that other world I inhabit,
that space that holds my life.
Here I'm in a magic place
learning once again to trace
the faces in the land
But everywhere I look I see
two young faces staring at me
staring with frightening intensity
as questions shape their minds.

They're the faces of twins
4 years old
faces I simply can't ignore
of new life come to mine.
Indu named for a holy river
Roshan for heat and light.

And when those faces catch my eye
I think of how they've changed my 'I'
I thrill to think, but nervously,
that I am three and three is me.

[1] Used as a title for a book by radical adult educators Myles Horton and Paolo Freire.
[2] A cave on a Blue Mountains property called Glastonbell that is often used for group meditations. This poem was written during a camp for undergraduate Social Ecology students at Glastonbell in March 1999.

References

Belenky, M., Clinchy, B., Goldberger, N. and Tarule, J. (1986) *Women's Ways of Knowing: The Development of Self, Voice and Mind*. New York: Basic Books.

Byrne-Armstrong, H. (1999) Dead certainties and local knowledge: Poststructuralism, conflict and narrative practices in radical/experiential education. PhD thesis, University of Western Sydney, Hawkesbury, NSW, Australia.

Hemery, C. (1995) Four shores. Thesis submitted as part requirement for a Graduate Diploma in Social Ecology, University of Western Sydney, Hawkesbury, NSW, Australia.

Lloyd, G. (1984) *The Man of Reason: 'Male' and 'Female' in Western Philosophy*. London: Methuen.

McKeon, R. (ed.) (1987) *Rhetoric: Essays in Invention and Discovery*. Woodbridge: Ox Bow.

Singer, P. (1995) *How Are We to Live? Ethics in an Age of Self-Interest*. Melbourne: Mandarin Books.

Ventura, M. (1995) The age of interruption. *Networker*, **19**(1), 22–26.

Waldrop, M. M. (1994) *Complexity: The Emerging Science at the Edge of Order and Chaos*. New York: Penguin.

Waring, M. (1996) *Three Masquerades: Essays on Equality, Work and Human Rights*. Sydney: Allen and Unwin.

Section Four

Glass ceilings and brick walls

12

Glass ceilings and brick walls: double disadvantage

Mary M Day

I'm hitting my head
Against a glass ceiling
A glass ceiling of gender-based discrimination
In the organizational hierarchy

I'm bashing my body
My spirit
My mind
Against a brick wall
A brick wall of methodological prescription
Prescribing the so-called 'mainstream'

Ouch
Sounds violent
'Tis violent
It hurts
I hurt
Ouch

I?
Who is 'I'?
Me!
She! A 'she' type person
A white She
Her
OK stop playing:
I *qua* poetic self
Constructing
Reproducing
I
My scholarly self
My feminist/critical/constructivist/postmodern
Scholarly self
My narratory self

And now back/forward to ceilings and walls
If not rooms of our own

Brick walls at least are easy to see
At least, they should be
Glass ceilings are invisible
Invisible to many
Invisible
To too many

The trick with glass ceilings
Is to catch the light
To see the light
On the glass
And then
Hey, you can see the light

But to *really* see
You need to crane your neck
To shift your position
To catch the reflection

To see
You need
To notice
Gender-based and
Taken-for-granted
Privileges

And it is a rare man
A man among men
Who acquaints himself
With his privileges
Who gazes in a mirror
Seeing his reflection

'Why,' says he
'Why would I bother?'
Precisely

Why?
Indeed
When wilful ignorance
Coupled with arrogance
Is so easy
Blissful even

Conscience not pricked
Really
Just pricks

And meanwhile
It is the men
Some men, most men
Who get tenure
And get promoted

And sooner
Or later
And preferable sooner
I learn
To stop hitting my head
To opt out
For a while
Out
Out of the game
'Cos it is a game
Only thing is
It is deadly to me
When I'm stuck there

So, it is less gung ho
More go slow
See the reflection
See what it means to me
See what it tells me
About me
About you

And it is us
Women
Who take on the educative role
I tried for years
To educate men
Why?
A martyr, perhaps?
I have stopped now
Sort of
Martyrdom really doesn't suit me

And so
A senior lecturer
I still be
He's an Aspro
What a pill
He's a Prof
Bigger still
And no better than me

And it is not just men
As all of us know
Some of our women colleagues
'Superiors' even
Have out-manned the men
How sad it is

I've learned to ride
To ride the injustice
The unfairness

And railing against it
Takes too much energy
Now I'm disabled
And I've learned
Recovery from workaholism
Well
Sort of
I am more wise
I pick the issues
I step back
Less gung ho
More slow

An ironic grin!!

Years later
I am planning
To apply for promotion
Slowly does it!

And now to brick walls
Strange things they are
Bricks of arrogance
Held tight
With mortared ignorance
Wilful ignorance/arrogance
Of methodological choice

'Cos it is a choice
Everyone makes
Knowingly
Or
Knowing it not

And the alternatives
Are just that
Alternatives
Except, of course
So-called 'mainstream' aka
Malestream
Functionalism
Positivism
Old and new
Are privileged true

'Alternative' is 'other'
Needing justification

When did you last notice
A 'mainstream' paper in which
The author justified
That methodological choice?

And if I feel
Yes
Feel
The violence of a Procrustean bed
When forced into no choice
Or justify your choice
I hurt
As limbs are stretched
Or cut off

And yet
I am lucky
There are journals
Just a couple
In my discipline of accounting
Yes
Accounting
Which are 'alternative' and 'critical'
Or at least, claim to be

Three years with one paper
Back and forth
Revision after revision
And in the paper I noticed
And commented on paradox
An editor
Slashed and burned to efface paradox
It was the last straw
I withdrew

Where do you go
When you are 'too critical'?

Supportive colleagues from other disciplines
Say
'Your discipline really needs you
And people like you'
Yes
But at what cost?
I ask myself

How can I survive?
I talk with supportive colleagues
I share stories with women colleagues
And yes 'bitch sessions' they are
And yet more than this
It is easier to see
When someone other than me
Is sucked in
We help each other
In many ways
Sewing circles

Swapping stitches
Creating new patterns
Helping to unpick
Assisting to create
Anew

We can and do
Still rail against the forced universal
Of funding application forms
Rail against the forced universal
Of most 'methods' subjects
Rail against the tyranny of numbers
Rail against the supremacy of numbers
But the world is changing
New voices are being heard
This text is just one
One of many
HURRAH

My pain
Your pain
Our pain
Not totally in vain

THE END

13

Breaking through with subjugated knowledges: pushing the boundaries of urban planning

Susan Thompson

Introduction

My account is one of backward beginnings, wrong ways of doing things, and problems I would rather not have had. Yet precisely because of these things, I think, the story is worth telling. (Krieger, 1991, p. 167)

'It is hard to be brave', said Piglet, sniffing slightly, 'when you're only a Very Small Animal'. Rabbit, who had begun to write very busily, looked up and said: 'It is because you are a very small animal that you will be Useful in the adventure before us'. (Hoff, 1993, p. iii, after Milne)

Smallness is an ironic quality. In Piglet's case it undermined his bravery in the face of adventure. For me, it challenged my passion for research and the way in which I used exclusively qualitative methods in an urban planning context. And yet it is the very quality of our Smallness that gives both Piglet and me the ability to contribute in our own unique and creative ways.

In this chapter I share my Smallness as a qualitative researcher in urban planning. And while mine is a tale of struggle and challenge, it is also a narrative of learning and inspiration, complexity and mystery, joy and excitement, and of growth and transformation, both in personal and professional terms. I tell my story because it is essential that we expose the personal difficulties encountered in the act of innovative and creative research, as well as debunking the mythology that scholarly inquiry is free from doubt, personal despair and chaos. It is also about declaring that researchers are people with feelings and experiences, as well as thinkers, writers and teachers. By adopting a reflexive stance as central to our practice, we can build up an enormously valuable collective resource upon which novice and experienced researchers can draw.

Although many people working in the social sciences privately discuss the idiosyncrasies, quirks and problems of doing research, public discussion and written accounts remain rare. The personal tends to be carefully removed from public statements: these are full of rational argument, careful discussion of academic points of dispute and frequently empty of any feeling of what the research process was actually like. (Stanley and Wise, 1979, p. 360)

In this chapter I focus on my doctoral research, which examined migrant women's meanings of home from a qualitative, subjective and contextual perspective. I discuss the manner in which I responded to the many questions and criticisms that I encountered, the unanswered questions that remain, and how this process strengthened and enhanced my thesis, as well as my determination and conviction to continue to practise as a qualitative researcher and hopefully to inspire others to follow.

Positioning the personal: who am I in this process?

I wish to suggest that the self is not a contaminant, but rather that it is key to what we know, and that methodological discussions might fruitfully be revised to acknowledge the involvement of the self in a positive way. (Krieger, 1991, pp. 29–30)

It is important at the outset of any writing to enunciate the assumptions that lie at the heart of the author's position. In my case they are grounded in personal, professional and academic experiences. The post-positivist context of contemporary research permits acknowledgment of its value-ladenness (Lather, 1986) and of the fact that it does not occur in a vacuum. Research is influenced at every stage by an individual's background and value system, as well as by the inquiry process itself.

Who I am in my work has been influenced by a multiplicity of experiences, both within and outside the academy. My educational background is in human geography, town planning and education, which in part explains my eclectic and interdisciplinary approach. I have always believed that adhering to one particular discipline will fragment understanding. I am also driven by a fascination with the relationship between people and place, having contemplated these issues for many years (Thompson, 1998). I have wondered about the qualities that make a place special and the factors that influence people's connection with their physical environment. I have also considered the role of daily interactions, the imagination and dreaming in creating a special place.

During the time I worked as a town planner, I often thought about the nature of neighbourhoods and domestic environments. From personal experience I knew that the home carried significant meaning, and yet this aspect hardly rated a mention in housing and neighbourhood policies. I wondered if this absence was in some way related to planning's preoccupation with the 'scientific', observable and tangible. Or was it to do with the discipline's reluctance to consider human emotions, dreams and aspirations? I was also conscious of being at odds with many of my (mostly male) colleagues, who did not universally share my belief that social issues were (and still are) just as important as other considerations in planning. Even though the need to consider social issues is enshrined in legislation, the long-standing separation of physical and social planning in Australia reinforces the latter's lesser status.

I have carried these professional interests and passions into the university where I now teach and research urban planning issues, particularly around difference and diversity. Much of my work is grounded in the ideology of feminism. This was the research philosophy that I adopted for my doctoral research.

> The overt ideological goal of feminist research is to correct both the 'invisi-
> bility' and the 'distortion' of female experience in ways relevant to ending
> women's unequal social position. This entails the substantive task of making
> gender a fundamental category for our understanding of the social order, 'to
> see the world from women's place in it'. (Callaway, 1981, in Lather, 1986,
> p. 68)

As a feminist researcher, I am motivated by a desire to enable women to speak from their lived experience in a way that does not objectify them. This means valuing the participants throughout and beyond the project. It also demands a methodological position that acknowledges the contextual and subjective.

My research philosophy is also grounded in the practice of reflection. For some this practice can be seen as 'doubting' the process, which is anathema in academe. However, for me it is central to any research endeavour. Reflecting on the responses to my doctoral research helped me to achieve a much greater understanding about who and what delineate the boundaries of my discipline, as well as what knowledge is deemed 'acceptable'. I was able to address issues such as: Who defines what is a 'legitimate' urban planning study in a changing world? Who dictates what methods can and cannot be used? Who determines what sort of knowledge is valued over any other, and what are the power structures that support the notion that 'objective' rationality is the only way of knowing?

I encountered students in seminars using positivist research who were never required to justify their approach, nor questioned about their method or the assumptions upon which it was based. Indeed, there was no acknowl-edgment that they were dealing with assumptions; these were givens. Conversely, I was often grilled about my method and its philosophical base, frequently patronized with comments such as 'women and the sub-urbs, how banal', or 'what has this got to do with town planning?'. Throughout these experiences I was encouraged by fellow qualitative researchers also struggling for legitimacy in their fields.

Reflecting on the process of research is often seen as something that is best done apart from the rigour and 'objectivity' of the academy. Accounts of the research experience are increasingly available (see, for example, Hertz, 1997), but they are still marginal to the mainstream methodological litera-ture. In my case, reflecting on the process of research has been instrumental to my understanding of the complexity of the issues with which I have been grappling. My story is about the struggle for legitimacy of qualitative research in urban planning, as much as it is about my individual path in undertaking the study. The fact that my method *was* such an issue meant that it was important to explore why this was the case.

The voices of challenge

I now turn to the research experience itself, and the challenges I faced in breaking through the traditional boundaries of knowledge in my discipline. The voices of challenge came in many forms and disguises. They were cloaked in reason, logic, objectivity, relevance and professionalism. They had something to say about my philosophical position, my subject matter, my use of language and my research methodology, including the analysis and theoretical interpretation.

Likewise, my responses came in many forms. Emanating from both emotional and intellectual knowing, they attempted to explain the reasons for my philosophical stance, choice of subject and methodology. In trying to provide these explanations, I have learnt the difficulties of crossing the conceptual bridge between positivism and a subjective, qualitative framework. The latter's valuing of other ways of knowing is particularly at odds with positivism's focus on intellectual understanding, logic and quantification. At times the negative feedback made me feel scared and lonely, as well as alienated from my discipline. I was a freak: on the margins. An outsider. Someone who was being 'difficult'. Ironically, I was often encouraged by those in other fields, who affirmed the relevance and importance of my contribution and expressed their disbelief that my work, particularly its philosophical and methodological bases, was indeed an issue. As a solo researcher, especially a doctoral candidate, constant voices of challenge and doubt are difficult to counter, even if one is confident of both the topic and the approach. However, the process of sharing and reflecting these experiences was enormously supportive, and ultimately pushed me beyond overwhelming self doubt to a belief in what I was doing, and consequently in my ability to complete. I believe that in reflecting more honestly about the research process, rather than pretending it is simple, ordered, straightforward and free of doubt, we stand to learn a great deal. This learning is not confined to improving our research techniques; rather it has the potential to break down the barriers between intellectual and emotional knowing. In turn, this is the only way that we will be able to begin to understand the intricate complexities of the social sciences and the contemporary research quandaries with which we grapple.

Challenges to my philosophical position

The problem ...
My exclusive use of the qualitative paradigm was fundamental to many critiques of my work. There was an assumption that, at best, such an unstructured approach should augment, not replace, quantitative research. Apart from the specifics of the methodology, which I discuss later, there was an underlying scepticism about a research paradigm that did not measure up to the standard tenets of positivism. There was also considerable difficulty with a process that was not set in concrete at the outset. Franck (1987, p. 61) discusses the dilemmas of qualitative researchers competing for funding:

> *... positivist approaches, including empiricism, are useful for seeking and receiving research grants because of their mandate to collect quantitative data in a way that is described and justified before the data collection begins.*

My feminist orientation to the research, to both its subject focus and methodology, was another primary target for challenge. I was frequently asked to define this philosophy and to justify why I had adopted a feminist position.

My response ...

As a social scientist, I operate from the assumption that there are different ways of doing research. The issue for me is one of appropriateness. Given that I was investigating the profound meaning of home, the usefulness of quantification techniques appeared extremely limited in this context. The choice of women as subjects also pointed to the need to examine different research methodologies that would access the intuitive, emotional and spiritual aspects inherent in women's ways of knowing (Belenky *et al.*, 1986). Franck (1989) was also helpful here, with her seven qualities that characterize feminine 'ways of knowing' and analysing, providing further methodological justification. These ways of knowing are based on the tenet of connection in women's relationships. They encompass (Franck, 1989, p. 203):

- an underlying sensitivity and connection to others, objects of knowledge, and the world
- a desire for inclusiveness, and to overcome opposing dualities
- a responsibility to respond to the needs of others, represented by an 'ethic of care'
- an acknowledgment of the value of everyday life and experience
- an acceptance of subjectivity as a strategy for knowing, and of feelings as part of knowing
- an acceptance and desire for complexity
- an acceptance of change and a desire for flexibility.

In planning research these qualities are rarely acknowledged, let alone heard or examined (see, for example, Sandercock and Forsyth, 1992). My data-gathering tools, principally in-depth interviews, acknowledged not only the validity of women's 'ways of knowing', but also the personal, contextual and holistic nature of existence. The approach gave me the flexibility to rework my initial question schedule in order to explore the unexpected, and to go back to my respondents, asking them to expand on issues and provide feedback on interpretations. To enable women to speak, I used lived experience as a key. Phenomenology, with its valuing of this experience, was critical.

> *What phenomenology can reveal about the imaginative meanings of our lived spaces is not nothing; it is potentially the greatest something which has been offered to those of us who wish to remain sensitive to the needs and desires which make our settlements truly human. (Stefanovic, 1985, p. 376)*

I found reference to the importance of using lived experience in the literature on home (for example, Saunders and Williams, 1988). I also considered that listening to women's everyday stories would help develop an understanding of gender differences. Encouraging women to tell their stories is particularly important in ethnic communities, where the policy of multiculturalism has encouraged a homogenizing of difference. Men have tended to speak for the whole group, perpetuating an acceptance of traditional social and power relationships (de Lepervanche, 1992).

By valuing what the migrant women told me and not imposing a predetermined set of questions on them, I was able to establish that loss was central to their concept of home as settlers in a new country. The development of my interviewee's trust, which took time and personal involvement, was essential here. Without her trust, there would not have been the level of in-depth sharing and reflections that I was privileged to witness. The women's story-telling process was a powerful vehicle for their considerations and allowed them to come to realizations that would have been impossible using a positivist survey technique. This is also the case in a current research project, where I am exploring changing meanings of home for people who have experienced the loss of a significant relationship.

The existence of seminal studies using qualitative approaches to examine meanings of home further justified my methodological choice. Rubbo (1981) links 'life history' with 'housing history' as a way of telling one's story and allowing social and personal meanings to emerge. Korosec-Serfaty (1984) discusses the importance of hidden places to the meaning of home; Pennartz (1986), atmosphere; and Maglin (1981), the kitchen. A major study investigating meanings of home for women living in Victoria also uses qualitative methods as the central investigative tool (Barclay *et al.*, 1991).

And yet, even though I was able to articulate logical reasons for my research philosophy, I found it hard to understand why I continued to hear voices of doubt and scepticism. Some comprehension did come from Caplan (1993, p. 55):

> ... *one prevalent attitude is that the presence of emotional content indicates the absence of academic and intellectual content. Women's studies . . . are often regarded as illegitimate offspring of academia, 'fuzzy' in methods, lacking in discipline and 'real content'.*

My position as a feminist influenced the decision to explore migrant women's meanings of home. From my general understanding of gender relations in society and from my knowledge of the planning system, I wanted to undertake research in a way that valued women. Because of the structuring of roles within society, women often believe that they do not have a great deal to offer policy-makers and academics. Statements such as 'I am only a housewife, how could I help?' serve to reinforce this myth. Together with her ethnicity, the migrant woman has been doubly disadvantaged. She has also been ignored in planning research, despite increasing levels of multiculturalism. The potentially empowering nature of research was another motivation. As a feminist, I wanted to use a method that had the potential to challenge the traditional, 'distant' relationship between researcher and researched.

This is not to say that in order to empower, research methodologies must emanate from a feminist perspective. The latter motivated my desire to select an approach that had such potential. Yet it was not easy, given the unequal sharing of power in my role as a university-educated Anglo-Celtic woman interviewing women from non-English speaking backgrounds, many with much lower levels of education. Also, my use of English as a first language was potentially problematic. However, these factors had to be balanced with other considerations. For example, in some communities, being an outsider can be an advantage. A member of the same community may be perceived as a potential informant to others within the group, resulting in the respondent being less open and honest. An outsider does not present the same threat. The fact that the women were able to speak about personal issues, even though they often reminded them of painful experiences, indicated to me that a degree of comfort was achieved between us. The length of interviews and their empowering nature, as expressed to me by the women, further validated my decision to use qualitative methods.

As a matter of course, I do not object to having to justify my philosophical stance, but I was at a loss to explain or understand why those undertaking more 'traditional', positivist studies were not so consistently challenged. Was it perhaps more than my feminist perspective that invited disapproval? Was there a concern about taking an integrated approach, bringing the personal, professional and academic together? The choice of topic was motivated by more than just intellectual curiosity. I wanted to research something that fascinated me and would contribute to my personal growth and understanding, not simply my intellect. Doing the project was not only about getting the required 'piece of paper'. Perhaps my critics had difficulty with a personal commitment to research, as well as with a project that focused on women. Or was the objection to an investigation that did not honour the traditional power relations between interviewer and interviewee?

It continues to disappoint me that there is little encouragement for those who attempt to push the boundaries of knowledge in creative and innovative ways. This is particularly the case in academia, where the traditional culture is individualistic and competitive. There are pockets of support, and I am thankful that I continue to find them, but my experience suggests that the degree of challenge and the level of justification required far surpass the demands on researchers doing more 'traditional' and less risky work.

Challenges to my subject for research

The problem ...
My subjects for research, women and home, were constantly under scrutiny. I was asked: Why only women? Surely men and children are important too? Some commentators expressed the view that, while the work was all very well, my interpretations did not sit comfortably with their meanings of home. This was particularly problematic, they asserted, when their experiences were situated in migrant households.

My response ...
Of course men and children are important! But the reality of research is that it is limited and must be focused. Any one project must have clearly defined boundaries. Despite the apparent reasonableness of this response (or did I miss something?) I was still challenged and, in extreme cases, accused of bias and antagonism toward the male of the species!

Logically, it was easy to defend my subject choice. Ethnicity did not feature in the literature on the meaning of home. Nor did a specific consideration of women migrants. Both are still hard to find. The relationship between policy and the intense personal attachment to home was, and still is, largely absent in the mainstream housing debate. So too was a considered analysis of multiculturalism in planning policy and practice. Llewellyn-Smith and Watson (1992, p. 78) confirmed my view here. This situation is slowly changing with the emergence of significant work on difference and diversity (see, for example, Fincher and Jacobs, 1998; Sandercock, 1998) as well as the research I have been conducting with colleagues in both planning and geography (Thompson *et al.*, 1998).

Nevertheless, when I was in the midst of my doctoral studies, the choice of migrant women and home was controversial. Upon reflection, I do not think that the intellectual component of my topic was such a problem. Rather, I believe it was the presence of a personal commitment and interest that may have been more of an issue. So while there were manifold justifications for the topic focus, there was objection to my attachment to studying women and home.

The notion that everyone has an experience of home is a difficult one too. I had fascinating conversations with a wide range of people, keen to share their meaning of home in a positive and encouraging way. It was those who interpreted what I was doing as a direct challenge to their conceptualizations that were disturbed by my findings. I endeavoured to counter their disquiet by explaining the boundaries of my research and the uniqueness of individual experience, together with the unifying themes that drew my interviewees' stories together.

Challenges to my methodology

The problem ...
The specifics of my methodological approach were constant targets for attack. The questions and comments raised included:

- Where are your hypotheses?
- What is your theoretical basis?
- What is your sample size? Is that representative?
- Can you replicate the research?
- What do you DO with all that data?
- The findings of this study are not generalizable.
- This form of research should be a precursor to the 'real' research using numerical and statistical analyses.
- This is subjective in the extreme and has no place in urban and regional planning.

My response ...
Within the qualitative or intensive paradigm, research questions focus the inquiry but do not exclude the possibility of other issues emerging and subsequently being explored as data collection and analysis proceed. In contrast to the positivist paradigm, research hypotheses are rarely formulated. My work was guided, but not solely defined, by a series of well thought out and comprehensive research questions (Thompson, 1996, pp. 15–16), ranging from the empirics to theorizing.

Nevertheless, the critical voices alleged illegitimacy. Hypotheses and theoretical positions validate the research process. Flexibility and theory grounded in data contrast so markedly that an approach where they are central is bound to be viewed with suspicion. So too is the inherent 'messiness' of qualitative research, especially the amount of data generated by in-depth interviews and reflective memos.

There is a potential to read too much or too little into the data. The fact that the researcher, rather than a statistical package, is the instrument of analysis brings the process into further disrepute. However, this subjectivity needs to be put into perspective when comparing the limitations of statistics in social research. The assumptions of positivists are rarely acknowledged, whereas good qualitative researchers are meticulous in explicating their value base and philosophical position. It is because we have become so enmeshed with the scientific that we take its assumptions as givens. This is certainly the case with the concept of generalizability.

The ability to generalize the results of positivist inquiry is frequently cited as one of its greatest strengths (Lincoln and Guba, 1985). Conversely, the inability to do the same with qualitative research is seen by some as a major weakness. The use of in-depth case studies is all very well, argue the critics, but what can they say about society at large, and how can a non-representative sample inform policy, theory and practice?

There are two issues to consider here. First, we need to question the notion of generalizability, given the unique and contextual nature of individual experience. The use of random sampling does not guarantee a representative group from which generalizations can be made. The notion of generalizability has been so highly valued that we have not critically looked at our ability to do this within the positivist framework or contemporary postmodern contexts. In attempting to generalize, one takes from the unique experience of the individual. Therefore, to generalize can, in some cases, be highly inaccurate (Lincoln and Guba, 1985, pp. 110–128).

The second aspect relates to the strength of in-depth and contextual understanding that is possible with qualitative research, compared with an ability to generalize. What is lost in the potential to generalize has to be weighed against the qualitative researcher's depth of understanding. In my study I found a heterogeneous experience, albeit with patterns of commonality. Accordingly, I would be sceptical of a large-scale survey that purported to find a homogeneous and highly generalizable set of concepts in this context.

Challenges to interpretations and applications

The problem . . .

A constant question about my research concerned its relevance to the discipline within which I was principally working. I was often asked, 'What does this have to do with town planning?'. Town planning, so the doubters declared, is concerned with broad issues, not the minutiae of everyday living. 'How can you contribute to policy with so few interviews?'; 'You say your research cannot be generalized, but surely this is necessary if you are to make a contribution to policy?'.

My response . . .

In arguing the relevance of home to town planning, I found many researchers across the globe who considered it an important topic in urban studies, particularly from the perspective of lived experience (see, for example, Saunders and Williams, 1988; Lawrence, 1989, 1991; Despres, 1991; Arias, 1993; Cooper Marcus, 1995).

At the time, the use of qualitative research was not widespread in town planning. I thought this odd, because planners are constantly making decisions about physical environments which impact on the daily lives of people. On the other hand, the absence of qualitative approaches was easier to understand, given the profession's preoccupation with the physical environment and the separation of this focus from social planning. Accordingly, it was hardly surprising that multicultural issues had not been on the Australian planning agenda. As Llewellyn-Smith and Watson (1992, p. 79) write:

> Given the structural separation in Australia between what is called social planning and what is called physical planning the likelihood of multicultural issues surfacing onto physical planning agendas seems low. This separation provides the context for understanding many of the urban and social problems which arise in Australian cities. Rather than physical planning being conceived as the provision of land, housing, roads, urban infrastructure for clear social ends, physical planning sometimes becomes an end in itself ...

Although the situation is slowly improving at both the theoretical level (Sandercock, 1998) and in local government practice (Thompson et al., 1998), my discussions with colleagues and students continue to confirm the discipline's reluctance to relinquish the primacy of physical planning. Those who expressed doubts that my doctoral research had relevance for town planning argued that planners should not be interested in the intimate relationship between individuals and their homes, nor in what migrants from non-English speaking backgrounds had to say about it. Further, the house was perceived as the domain of architects.

The use of detail was seen as foreign to the concerns of town planning. My critics argued that interpretations of the 'big picture' were the only relevant data for policy review. And yet, the assessment of detail is central to the development control process. I wondered whether the rejection of detail as a legitimate concern of the discipline constituted a devaluing of the day-to-day work of the planner. In my experience these tasks are always viewed as much less prestigious than strategic or long-range planning, particularly at the regional and state levels.

I found it useful to look at existing planning policies in relation to the tension between detail and broader perspectives. An example is urban consolidation policy. The meaning of home, particularly the intense emotional attachment to the house and garden, is largely ignored, as are multicultural considerations. It is necessary to ask why, given the community's reluctance to adopt 'consolidated' lifestyles. So much of the literature confirmed the need to take meanings of home into account. My research, which added the extra dimension of multiculturalism, provided further validation.

My inquiry illuminated patterns of experience, providing an understanding of the relationship between experience and meanings of home. By extrapolating from the patterns, it is possible to gain new insights into policy. Even if one accepts the argument that policy cannot change as the result of a single qualitative study, the potential of comparative work cannot be dismissed. It can be used to compare and contrast qualitative findings across time and contexts, thereby constructing an in-depth and detailed understanding of social issues.

Challenges to my language

The problem ...
My use of personal pronouns and 'easy-to-understand' language or plain English was criticized by some in the academy.

My response ...
The adoption of personal pronouns in reporting my work was carefully considered in the broader context of qualitative research. Richards (1990), an experienced and respected qualitative researcher, rejects terms such as 'respondent' and 'researcher' because they imply a one-way model of interviewing and a distancing of the author from the process of research. Swanson-Kauffman (1986, p. 59) argues that use of the third person is inappropriate in qualitative work, given its philosophical base:

> *Not only did I value my informants' capacity to teach me about their reality, I also had to believe in my capacity to break into that reality, reflect on it, make it my own, and ultimately share my lived experience as a qualitative . . . researcher.*

The use of the third person can give a misleading impression of the researcher as an unbiased, impassive observer with no influence on the research process or its outcome. In choosing to write in the first person, I was also influenced by Krieger (1991), who argues strongly for more of the self in both social science and its writing. In what I can only describe as inspirational and groundbreaking writing, she relates her own struggle to bring the personal into social science inquiry. She speaks in the first person, challenging the traditional view that the self 'contaminates' research:

> *The problem we need worry about is not the effect of an observer's inner self on evidence from the outside world, but the ways that the traditional dismissal of the self may hinder the development of each individual's unique perspective. (Krieger, 1991, p. 30)*

In my writing I also tried to present my ideas clearly and, as far as possible, in plain English. Whilst this practice is being adopted within government, it is not a priority in universities (National Ideas Summit, 1990). As an academic I have often felt pressure to conform to a particular style, but have resisted in the belief that it is important for research to be accessible to the broader community. Some of the pressure I experienced came from comparing my expression with that of so-called 'postmodern' authors. I was concerned that my work would not be perceived as academically credible if it did not adopt this style. I was worried that clarity and ease of understanding would be perceived as simplistic and naive. My decision to reject this way of communicating was reinforced by Garreau's (1991, p. 485) impression of some postmodern writing:

> *Sadly, the term 'postmodern' is also all too often wrapped like a protective cloak around writing that mistakes incomprehensibility for profundity.*

I was also inspired by Krieger (1991, p. 36):

> *We are encouraged to speak in generally acceptable styles, rather than to speak in ways that are our own. The ability to speak from within takes nurturance. It requires the use of one's own words rather than the use of currently fashionable words in one's discipline ...*

In addition, I was mindful of the subject of my thesis. I wanted the work to have the potential to be read by non-academics, members of the ethnic communities I was researching, and practising urban planners. It is in such a context of accessibility that Massey (1991, p. 34) advocates 'democratic writing':

> *Much writing in and about postmodernism verges on the pretentious, and on occasions the virtually incomprehensible to those not in a {fairly small} group.*

The irony, which is not lost on Massey, is the way in which such postmodern writing alienates and excludes the very groups that postmodernism claims to be bringing into 'fuller appreciation' (p. 32). They are immediately marginalized in terms of their understanding, and the power inequities between researcher and researched are further reinforced. Plain English can be used to help research participants better understand the outcomes of an investigation. Other methods of returning the research to the participants can also be employed to facilitate understanding (see e.g. Roberts, 1984).

I also used gender-neutral language. This choice was based on my feminist values and the argument that language has power that can perpetuate women's invisibility and inequity. In addition, the use of sexist language has long been rejected as unacceptable in government and academic publications (Australian Government Publishing Service, 1988).

The challenge of representation: how can I speak for these women?

The problem ...

For some time now there has been a considerable and long overdue debate about representation, or the ethics of being able to speak for the other. This is and was very pertinent to my research, given that I am a non-migrant, white, Anglo-Celtic woman researching migrant women from non-English speaking backgrounds. On a number of occasions I was rightly challenged about my position and asked to explain my 'presence'.

My response ...

Writing on the politics of making films about Aborigines, Marcia Langton (1993, p. 27), an Aboriginal woman, offers some timely reflections about representations of indigenous Australians. She highlights problems of objectifying, stereotyping and writing on behalf of the 'other' without declaring one's own background. Although specifically addressing indigenous issues, her message is applicable to other situations of representation:

> *There is a naive belief that Aboriginal people will make 'better' representations of us, simply because being Aboriginal gives 'greater' understanding. This belief is based on an ancient and universal feature of racism: the assumption of the undifferentiated 'Other'. More specifically, the assumption is that all Aborigines are alike and equally understand each other, without regard to cultural variation, history, gender, sexual preference and so on. It is a demand for censorship: there is a 'right' way to be Aboriginal, and any Aboriginal film or video producer will necessarily make a 'true' representation of 'Aboriginality'. (Langton, 1993, p. 27)*

Problems occur when the person making the representation (in Langton's case, the film-maker; in mine, the researcher) objectifies that which is being studied, distancing and separating researcher and researched, film-maker and filmed. Awareness of this possibility is critical, as is the understanding that all research is an interpretive act grounded in a particular perspective.

My work on migrant women's meanings of home can, in the end, represent only *my* interpretation of the stories I heard. As much as I tried to be true to the women's lived experience, there was a point where I had to take the data, essentialize themes and interpret interrelationships through my perspective as a middle-class, educated, feminist woman:

> *... we have to be willing to work across all our differences ... our work must necessarily address the issue of intersubjectivity with the explicit recognition of two points.*
>
> *1. ... we are engaged in an interpretive act ... the double hermeneutic of interpreting others' interpretations of what they are doing.*
>
> *2. ... we enter into this interpretive act from what has been variously referred to as a 'politics of position' or 'politics of location' ... that is, those places and spaces we inherit and occupy which frame our lives in very specific and concrete ways ... (Peake, 1993, p. 420)*

Negotiating the doubting voice: criticism as positive challenge

In this final section, I provide some practical suggestions for qualitative researchers working in overly critical and non-supportive environments. These come directly from my experiences and are offered in a positive and supportive context.

First, it is important to see the critic as an ally. Negative and judgmental comments are valuable data, which are not to be feared or shunned. Welcome them and use them as part of your reflexive practice. Interrogate the critique. What is it saying about your research and the discipline within which you are working? What positions of power are represented, and how does your work challenge them?

Second, learn how to be a rigorous qualitative researcher. Sloppy research is bad research, irrespective of who conducts it and the paradigm within which it is situated. Ensure that your practice stands up to the measures of trustworthiness for qualitative research (see, for example, Lincoln and Guba, 1985). Learn from the leaders in the field and encourage others to do likewise.

Third, seek out support in as many ways as you can. Talk to all sorts of people. Do not discount unlikely sources of help. Join a qualitative support group. Set up your own if you cannot find an established one. Encourage others to participate, and do not be bound by your own discipline. 'Talk' on the Internet and explore opportunities for interactive bulletin boards where researchers share ideas, struggles and victories.

Fourth, believe in yourself and your work and realize that you cannot please everyone! Doing innovative and unorthodox research presents a challenge to those around you. They are confronted with questions about who they are and what they are doing. This can be uncomfortable, and may result in unfair and biased criticism dressed up as reasoned argument. Do not be offended. Examine the critique for what it can provide and if it emanates from ignorance and fear, move on and seek support from those unperturbed by your approach.

Fifth, get your credentials as a researcher. Whether we like it or not, there is power in having that 'piece of paper'. If you want to work in academia, qualifications are important. With them you can rise to positions of power and influence and begin to change the system from within, legitimizing different research practices and paradigm shifts.

Finally, actively encourage qualitative research training in your discipline. Education breaks the influence of ignorance. Go out there and spread the word. Offer interesting courses in qualitative methods. Teach students how to conduct rigorous qualitative inquiry. Demonstrate the power of the method to enable in-depth understanding of the social and cultural world.

Conclusion

Qualitative research is difficult to undertake, and demands personal commitment and passion. It is a testing and personally challenging process, particularly for those of us working in disciplines where the approach is viewed with scepticism. For those who question orthodox conceptualizations of power and order, there are even greater hurdles. The importance of establishing support networks is paramount, as is the development of rigorous practice and a belief in what one is doing. By sharing our experiences of carrying out qualitative research we empower each other. We learn from our mistakes, the difficulties and challenges we face, and our responses to criticism, whether justifiable or unfair. We need to speak openly about our inner doubt and alienation, as well as acknowledge the intellectual, emotional and experiential knowing that we bring to the research act. We do not have to avoid or fear the critic or cynic. My experience shows how these voices pushed me to believe in the work I was doing, ultimately reinforcing my conviction of the importance of qualitative research in urban planning and the decision to continue researching in this paradigm. I found strengths I never knew were mine, and, in sharing my story, I hope someone else will be encouraged to go on and do likewise. The outcome is a creative and exciting journey, one I would not have missed for anything.

References

Arias, E. G. (ed.) (1993) *The Meaning and Use of Housing: International Perspectives, Approaches and Their Applications*. Aldershot: Avebury.

Australian Government Publishing Service (1988) *Style Manual for Authors, Editors and Printers*, 4th edn. Canberra: AGPS.

Barclay, L., Johns, L., Kennedy, P. and Power, K. (1991) *Speaking of Housing ... A Report on a Consultation with Victorian Women on Housing for the Minister for Planning and Housing*. Melbourne: Ministerial Advisory Committee on Women and Housing and Women in Supportive Housing.

Belenky, M., Clinchy, B., Goldberger, N. and Tarule, J. (1986) *Women's Ways of Knowing*. New York: Basic Books.

Caplan, P. (1993) *Lifting a Ton of Feathers: A Woman's Guide to Surviving in the Academic World*. Toronto: University of Toronto Press.

Cooper Marcus, C. (1995) *House as a Mirror of Self: Exploring the Deeper Meaning of Home*. Berkeley: Conari Press.

de Lepervanche, M. (1992) Working for the man: migrant women and multiculturalism. In *Gender Relations in Australia: Domination and Negotiation* (K. Saunders and R. Evans, eds), pp. 82–96. Sydney: Harcourt Brace Jovanovich.

Despres, C. (1991) The meaning of home: literature review and directions for future research and theoretical development. *The Journal of Architectural and Planning Research*, **8**(2), 96–115.

Fincher, R. and Jacobs, J. (eds) (1998) *Cities of Difference*. New York: Guilford Press.

Franck, K. (1987) Phenomenology, positivism, and empiricism as research strategies in environment–behaviour research and design. In *Advances in Environment, Behaviour, and Design*, Vol. 1 (E. Zube and G. Moore, eds), pp. 59–67. New York: Plenum Publishing.

Franck, K. (1989) A feminist approach to architecture: acknowledging women's ways of knowing. In *Architecture – A Place for Women* (E. P. Berkeley and M. McQuaid, eds), pp. 201–216. Washington: Smithsonian Institute Press.

Garreau, J. (1991) *Edge City: Life on the New Frontier*. New York: Anchor Books.

Hertz, R. (ed.) (1997) *Reflexivity and Voice*. Thousand Oaks: Sage.

Hoff, B. (1993) *The Te of Piglet*. London: Mandarin.

Korosec-Serfaty, P. (1984) The home from attic to cellar. *Journal of Environmental Psychology*, **4**, 303–321.

Krieger, S. (1991) *Social Science and the Self: Personal Essays on an Art Form*. New Brunswick: Rutgers University Press.

Langton, M. (1993) *Well, I Heard it on the Radio and I Saw it on the Television. . . .* North Sydney: Australian Film Commission.

Lather, P. (1986) Issues of validity in openly ideological research: between a rock and a soft place. *Interchange*, **17**(4), 63–84.

Lawrence, R. (1989) Houses and people in context: a conceptual model. *Architecture Australia*, **44**, 44–50.

Lawrence, R. (1991) The meaning and use of home. *The Journal of Architectural and Planning Research*, **8**(2), 91–95.

Lincoln, Y. and Guba, E. (1985) *Naturalistic Inquiry*. Beverly Hills: Sage.

Llewellyn-Smith, J. and Watson, S. (1992) Issues in cross-cultural planning. *Australian Planner*, **30**(2), 78–80.

Maglin, N. B. (1981) Kitchen dramas. *Heresies II*, **3**(3), 42–46.

Massey, D. (1991) Flexible sexism. *Environment and Planning D: Society and Space*, **9**, 31–57.

National Ideas Summit (1990) *Unlocking and Academies*. Sydney: Australian Council for the Arts.

Peake, L. (1993) 'Race' and sexuality: challenging the patriarchal structuring of urban social space. *Environment and Planning D: Society and Space*, **11**(4), 415–432.

Pennartz, P. (1986) Atmosphere at home: a qualitative approach. *Journal of Environmental Psychology*, **6**, 135–153.

Richards, L. (1990) *Nobody's Home: Dreams and Realities in a New Suburb*. Melbourne: Oxford University Press.

Roberts, H. (1984) Putting the show on the road: dissemination of research findings. In *Social Researching: Politics, Problems and Practice* (C. Bell and H. Roberts, eds), pp. 199–212. London: Routledge and Kegan.

Rubbo, A. (1981) Housing histories: a way of understanding the social and personal meaning of the domestic environment. *Heresies II*, **3**(3), 39–41.

Sandercock, L. (1998) *Towards Cosmopolis*. London: John Wiley.

Sandercock, L. and Forsyth, A. (1992) A gender agenda: new directions for planning theory. *Journal of the American Planning Association*, **58**(1), 49–59.

Saunders, P. and Williams, P. (1988) The constitution of home: towards a research agenda. *Housing Studies*, **3**(2), 81–93.

Stanley, L. and Wise, S. (1979) Feminist research, feminist consciousness and experiences of sexism. *Women's Studies International Quarterly*, **2**, 359–374.

Stefanovic, I. L. (1985) Phenomenological insights to guide the design of housing. *Ekistics*, **307**, 375–378.

Swanson-Kauffman, K. (1986) A combined qualitative methodology for nursing research. *Advances in Nursing Science*, **8**(3), 58–69.

Thompson, S. (1996) Women's stories of home: meanings of home for ethnic women living in established migrant communities. Unpublished PhD thesis, The University of Sydney, NSW, Australia.

Thompson, S. (1998) Editorial. *Urban Policy and Research*, **16**(1), 4–5.

Thompson, S., Dunn, K., Burnley, I., Murphy, P. and Hanna, B. (1998) *Multiculturalism and Local Governance: A National Perspective*. NSW Department of Local Government, Ethnic Affairs Commission, University of New South Wales, Sydney, NSW, Australia.

14

Dangerous knowledge – the politics and ethics of research

Moira Carmody

> *When sociologists do research, they inevitably take sides for or against parti-*
> *cular values, political bodies and society at large. That is they act as agents of*
> *the state, for interest groups or for themselves. In so doing, they take sides, for*
> *it is impossible to do value neutral research. (Denzin, 1989, p. 248)*

A recognition of the political nature of all social science research has
increasingly emerged since the late 1980s (e.g. Guba and Lincoln, 1989;
Reinharz, 1992; Punch, 1994). By 'politics' I mean, like Punch (1994, p.
84), everything from the micropolitics of personal relations to the culture
and resources of university research units and the powers and policies of
government and individual settings where research takes place. In extending
this concept further I turn to Foucault (1984, cited Rabinow, 1984, pp. 291–
292):

> *When one speaks of power people immediately think of political structure, a*
> *government, a dominant social class, the master and the slave, and so on. I am*
> *not thinking of this at all when I speak of relations of power. I mean that in*
> *human relationships, whether they involve verbal communication ... or amor-*
> *ous, institutional or economic relationships, power is always present: I mean a*
> *relationship in which one person tries to control the conduct of the other. So I*
> *am speaking of relations that exist at different levels, in different forms: these*
> *power relations are mobile, they can be modified, they are not fixed once and*
> *for all.*

Like all areas of knowledge production, power relations are embedded in
every aspect of the research process (Pearce, 1993). This includes the way the
research question is constructed, the topic to be studied, the people or issue
being explored, the biography and relations among researchers, the values
of the funding body and other actors involved in the particular project, and
the methodology chosen by the researcher. For me, speaking about sexual
and physical violence to women and children, through research, policy,
writing or teaching, is an act of resistance to community denial and victim
blaming and therefore highly political. I consciously 'choose sides'.

In thinking about writing this chapter, it occurred to me that it would be
hard to draw an arbitrary line around researching intimate violence as a
separate activity. This would have created an artificial boundary or brick
wall around what I see, feel and do. Over the last 25 years I have held a
number of different roles located in multiple sites, including community
health, hospital, sexual assault service, central office of state bureaucracy,

and tertiary education. Much of my work in these areas involves resisting the dominant beliefs and practices about sexual and physical violence[1] and attempting to provide space for alternative discourses to be heard. My work regarding intimate violence has taken many forms; all have been imbued with a commitment to the feminist project. Re-search(ing) has been a key aspect of all of these activities, and is woven into the fabric of my professional life. This awareness challenged me to consider how I currently conceptualize research.

Inherent in my reflections was an assumption that I was thinking of *social* research. Gilbert (1994, p. 18) suggests that 'there are three major ingredients in social research, the construction of theory, the collection of data, and no less important, the design of methods for gathering data'. This is one approach, but in focusing purely on the steps of the research process it fails to bring to life my feeling for research. My experience of research is primarily as a qualitative researcher and I recognize that research, expanding on Denzin and Lincoln's (1994, p. 3) comments, is an interactive process shaped by my personal history, biography, gender, social class, sexuality, ethnicity and ability, as well as those elements in the people in the setting. These elements therefore shape who I am as a researcher, what I choose to research and how.

Absent from many written accounts of research are the dilemmas, politics and ethical challenges that face researchers in the field. Punch (1994) reports a personal communication from Van Maanen arguing that this is because there is to date no genre or narrative convention in which researchers own up to how they have resolved these issues in the field. Further, Punch (1994) suggests that traditionalists tend to eschew 'politics'. However, Shakespeare, Atkinson and French (1993) suggest there is a developing literature of reflective research accounts. They argue that there is general agreement amongst many social researchers that knowledge is socially and culturally constructed. This means that the researcher and the researcher's actions are part of that process, and should therefore be subject to self-reflection. In this chapter I hope to contribute to challenging the silences about the politics and ethics of research through a reflexive and critical analysis of one research project for which I was chief investigator. I do this recognizing the crisis of representation confronting qualitative researchers in the postmodern period (Denzin, 1997). This project involved a full cast of players with different experiences and possible meanings of the same events. Mine is only one of many possible stories.

I have responded to this crisis of (re)presentation by heeding Denzin's (1997) invitation to pursue alternative ways of presenting research, and I have applied the politics and ethics of research by using the metaphor of a dramatic play. Speaking the unspeakable about intimate violence is a play of many acts in which many voices compete for space on the private and public stage. The characters and the action in any research project move from scene to scene, while twists and turns and shifting power relations are encountered between the actors. The following eleven-act drama script uses excerpts from research documents, conversations and actions between players, and reflections on behind-the-scenes action to highlight some of the critical moments in a research project which explored how vulnerable children and their families were treated in a general district hospital's Emergency

Department. The names of all the characters except my own are fictitious. I follow this with an analysis of issues raised by that research project, suggesting how awareness of those issues might be useful in negotiating other critical moments in qualitative research.

The play: *Dangerous Knowledge*

The characters (in order of appearance):

Moira Carmody: Senior Lecturer University of Western Sydney; Leading character and chief research investigator
Kate McFeast: Co-researcher, Child Protection Specialist for a health service, PhD student of Moira Carmody
Mary Smith: Co-researcher, PhD student of Moira Carmody
The Children and their Families who used the Health Service: Present throughout but not always visible
University Ethics Committee Members: Offstage
Commonwealth Department of Community and Health Services: Offstage
Mr Grey: Manager of District Health Service
Health workers employed in the Health Service: Present through their actions recorded in the medical files
Ms Senior: Manager of Area Health Service
Ms Junior: Representative of District Health Service
Mr Law: Legal Advisor, Area Health Service
Miss Cratt: Representative of the Commonwealth Department of Community and Health Services

Act 1. Anticipation and desire – 'the tender'

Characters: Moira
Setting: Home, Saturday morning paper, tea and toast

Commonwealth Department of Health and Family Services
INVITATION TO TENDER

National Council for the Prevention of Child Abuse Research Grants
... The Council is seeking submissions from appropriately qualified individuals and organizations to undertake research projects in the area of child abuse and neglect. The projects are to focus on one or both of the following topics:

● The Evaluation of Intervention Programmes
● The Evaluation of Preventative Programmes.

Special consideration will be given to high quality proposals on these two topics which also include:

● the views of clients
● the needs of Indigenous Australians.

. . . Closing date for submissions is 4pm on Friday 26 June, 1998

(Excerpt from call for tenders from *Sydney Morning Herald*, May, 1998)

Moira: This looks interesting ... Who else would be interested? ... Who has the other skills needed to complete the task? ... What do they actually want? ... What about Kate and Mary? I must ring them and ask them to have a look ...

Act 2. 'Writing the script' for the research bid: 'Building and evaluating child friendly preventative health services'

Characters: Moira, co-researchers Kate and Mary (both PhD students of Moira)

Setting: University office

> The purpose of this study is to evaluate the impact of an Area Child Protection Strategy in promoting a child-friendly and prevention-focused health service. The study will assess the medical records of all children presenting to the Emergency Department at one local hospital, before and after the implementation of the strategy. Locally developed policies that focus on prevention will be evaluated and compared against the findings of the medical record audit. This will provide a framework for ongoing evaluation which has national application. (Moira, Kate and Mary, Excerpt from the tender bid application)

Act 3. 'Do no harm' – Ethics Committee

Characters: Moira, University Ethics Committee members (offstage)

> If the file audit reveals any families in which inadequate response occurred by the health worker then two actions will follow. If it is believed that a child remains in a situation where they are vulnerable to child abuse a retrospective notification will be made to the Department of Community Services. Secondly, the system failure will be brought to the attention of the Area Health Service to reduce the chance of similar incidents reoccurring. Individual staff members will not be identified. (Moira, excerpt from University Ethics Committee application)

University of Western Sydney, Hawkesbury
Human Research Ethics Committee

12 October 1998

Memo to: Moira Carmody

Re: Ethics Application No 98:xxx

'Building and Evaluating Child Friendly Preventative Health Services'

I am pleased to inform you that the Human Research Ethics Committee has granted full ethics approval for your project ...

(Excerpt from University Ethics Committee approval)

Act 4. Getting a backer

> The Minister for Community Services, the Hon. Warren Truss MP, has approved funding for the research project 'Building and evaluating child

friendly preventative health services'. (Letter from the Commonwealth Department, 10 December 1998)

Act 5. Choosing the 'scene' for investigation

Characters: Moira, Kate, Mr Grey (District Health Manager)
Action: At the request of a specific District Health Service a meeting was held to negotiate access to the site and the process to be followed in obtaining medical records. A copy of the funding application and Ethics Committee application and approval was provided to Mr Grey.

Act 6. Rehearsals – bringing the study characters to life

Characters: Kate, Mary, Moira, children and their families, health workers
Action: *(Main stage)* data gathering at the health service by Kate and Mary
(Off stage) Moira facilitates meetings among research team members, reviews problems, prepares interim reports for funding body.

Act 7. Dangerous knowledge – writing up the data analysis and findings

An analysis of the findings indicate no significant improvement in the management of children who may be vulnerable to child abuse and who presented to the District Health Service Emergency Department in the two time periods of sampling. While the total number of children who met the screening tool requirements was small at 51 in total, the detailed analysis provides insight into how children and young people are both assessed and treated ...

... children under four years constituted the highest numbers of the presentations and a high percentage of the children were males ... The lack of information regarding the cultural background of children presenting to the Emergency Department can only hamper attempts to provide culturally sensitive services ...

... However the voices of younger children were found to be completely absent in the medical files. This is despite the research findings of the last ten years that clearly indicate that children as young as three can and should be consulted about their own lives ...

... Accidents, medical presentations, assault, burns and death were the major categories of presenting problems. While accidents and medical presentations may be attributed to a range of factors other than child abuse, a systematic social assessment of these children would have made it clearer if further action was required. Particularly concerning was the number of serious assaults which were indicative of family problems and received no further investigation. The two unexplained deaths, of boys two months and twelve months of age, raise serious questions about the health staff's awareness of their legal and professional responsibilities ...

... The medical file audit demonstrated that there were significant gaps in the information recorded on medical records, which indicate a lack of awareness

of both the Area Child Protection Guidelines and in some cases the Department of Health requirements to notify suspicions of child abuse and neglect to the Department of Community Services. In most cases health workers failed to be explicit about their decision-making processes. This is particularly important in cases where a child presents with an injury ...

... The introduction of the Area Child Protection Guidelines was preceded by training of key health staff. A rolling programme covering all of the mandatory information for health workers was devised and run in the District Health Service to ensure that all Emergency staff received training. This included the provision of work-based training modules provided at times suitable for all staff including night staff which was provided at 5 and 6 am. The attendance at the training was the highest in the Area at over 90 per cent ...

... This research further demonstrates that there are limitations to top-down policy implementation. Policy will be interpreted differently at every level of health service that is involved. In this study, despite clear policy and procedures supported by a high level of training of front-line staff, Emergency Department staff did not comply with policy directions. It would also seem that the guidelines required staff to shift ground from a purely medical model of health care delivery to incorporate a social model of health. This is a significant contrast in paradigms for staff in which fast and accurate medical assessment is the focus in an Emergency Department ...

... The findings also provide some insight into the complexities of providing public health care where the Area Health Service is fully government funded and subcontracts care to private providers. This market-driven approach to health care is underpinned by a belief in choice. In practice this may mean that private health care providers believe they have a choice in whether they follow Area or State Health Department policy directives. Indeed contracts between Area Health Services and private providers may allow them flexibility in following policy directives if they have resource implications. This raises significant issues about access and equity for the general public to a full health care system. In relation to the care of vulnerable children and their families it provides a potential way of avoiding taking legal and moral responsibility for protecting children. (Excerpts from the Final Research Report, 1999)

Act 8. Tension in the 'company'

Characters: Moira, Kate, Mary

(Stage left)

Mary: Why aren't I involved in feeding back to the Area Health Service? I'm feeling excluded ... Moira, you and Kate are leaving me out of this ...

(Stage right)

Kate: What is Mary on about? I'm there in my Area role as child protection advisor ... I wish she'd get a grip ... Moira, sort it out please ...

(Centre stage)

Moira: God, what is going on with these two? I thought I'd explained to Mary that Kate is there as an Area person and I'm there representing the research team as chief investigator ... Why is Mary getting so wound up? I've asked her to come in to have a meeting about it all but she seems to be too busy at present ... I wonder what is going on between Mary and Kate? What should I do? If I can't resolve this it could really jeopardize the project.

Act 9. Showtime – reporting back to stakeholders

Characters: Moira, Kate in Area Child Protection Role, Ms Senior (Area Health Manager), Ms Junior (Representative of District studied), Mr Laws (Area Health Legal Advisor)

Action: A copy of the final report was sent by Moira to the Area and District staff two days prior to the report back session. Chief Investigator summarizes the main findings and discusses the recommendations of the study. Area Health Manager requests response in writing from District within two weeks. District representative says little apart from indicating the District will be refuting the methodology but will not state in what way or why.

Act 10. The critics' reviews

Characters: Moira, Mr Grey (Manager, District Health Service)
Setting: University office of Moira
Action: Telephone rings.

Scene 1

Caller: This is Mr Grey from the District Health Service. I've been requested by my Executive to inform you that we intend to take legal action regarding the research you just completed on our service. We strongly dispute the methodology used.

Moira: What in particular is a problem?

Mr G: We don't see why my name and the name of the District Health Service is in the report and I am very annoyed that you did not show me a draft of the report before you presented it to the Area Health Service.

Moira: When we negotiated access to the site and set up the research which you were very keen for us to do, you did not request a draft. Anyhow what difference would that have made? Are you suggesting I would have changed my research findings?

Mr G: I don't see why it was necessary to name me. Anyhow I need to know how we can access the data you collected so we can check the truth of your claims. We will do this legally if necessary.

Moira: The data is the property of the funding body, the university and myself. If you have any enquiries about this I suggest you talk to the Pro-Vice Chancellor of Research. Despite the concerns you raise I hope the District will still consider the very serious findings and take steps to implement the recommendations.

Mr G: What is the phone number of the person in the research office I need to talk to?

Scene 2 (some months later)

Mr G: I am still concerned about the research you carried out identifying our service. What are you intending to do with the report? How widely has it been distributed?

Moira: The report was written for the Area Health Service, your service and the funding body. Any publications will not name your service or the Area.

Mr G: Are you willing to write a letter to that effect? And what about the funding body?

Moira: I can't speak for the funding body but I'm willing to confirm what I said in writing.

Mr G: I would appreciate that.

Moira: What is the District doing about implementing the recommendations of the research?

Mr G: We are implementing an action plan in relation to the findings. Will you send me the letter as soon as you can.

Moira: I'll send it today.

Act 11. The final act?

Characters: Moira, Miss Cratt (Funding Body representative)
Setting: University office of Moira
Action: Telephone call to Canberra.

Moira: It has been over four months since I submitted the revised final report and I have heard nothing from the Council. Could you tell me where things are up to, what the Council intends to do with the report?

Ms C: The National Council has looked at your final report. We consider it was an excellent report and raises a number of major issues of concern. However due to the sensitivity of the issues they have decided not to publish it but to use it for internal departmental advice.

Moira: I would appreciate it if you could send me a letter explaining that.

Four months later the letter has not arrived.

To be continued . . .

Reflections on dangerous knowledge

The above 'drama' highlights a series of critical moments in the development of one research project, and how power relations are embedded in all aspects of the research process. While not all research projects consist of so many fraught 'acts', researching sensitive topics such as child abuse and sexual violence may challenge the dominant culture's views of the issue or threaten stakeholders' perceptions of the work they do. This research study draws attention to the political perils and ethical pitfalls of actually carrying out research (Punch, 1994). An analysis of the behind the scenes action suggests three areas for reflection: researching a sensitive topic, negotiating relationships, and the politics of negative findings.

Researching a sensitive topic

A simple definition of *sensitive research* would be research that potentially poses a substantial threat to those who are or have been involved in it (Lee, 1993, p. 4). In particular, Lee's definition of political threat seems most useful in reflecting on this research project. Lee suggests that research can be problematic when it impinges on political alignments, arguing for a broad definition of 'political' that considers the vested interests of powerful people or institutions or the exercise of coercion or domination. Researching physical and sexual violence of women and children from a critical perspective potentially challenges the vested interests of the dominant culture concerning attitudes and beliefs about women and children. Until the early 1970s, community awareness and an organized government policy response to the issue of intimate violence were limited (Carmody, 1992). The success of feminist campaigns over the last 20 years in placing sexual and physical violence on the agenda of the state has resulted in significant social policy reform in Australia. Reforms have challenged community and government beliefs that intimate sexual violence is a private matter that has no place in the public work of the state (Carmody and Carrington, 2000). The area of child abuse has also received greater personal and professional attention since the mid-1960s as a result of work done by pediatricians and child advocates (Helfer and Kempe, 1976; Parton, Thorpe and Wattam, 1997). Over the ten years following the 1989 United Nations Convention on the Rights of the Child, there has been a growing recognition of the need to develop strategies to include children in decisions that affect them (James and Prout, 1990; Rayner, 1991; Hallett, 1993; Garbarino, 1995). Public exposure of the reality of violence against women and children has challenged societal assumptions about interpersonal relationships. In particular, it has revealed the insidious nature of violence which is a daily reality for many women and children, and the isolation and individual self-blame that are key features of the issue. Resisting the power of violence to shape intimate relationships becomes a political act. It is therefore implicitly necessary to 'take sides'. By choosing to research in this area, I aim to challenge the existing power relations and dominant cultural discourses about women and children.

The child-friendly research project was designed to assess health workers' responses to vulnerable children and their families who presented to an

Emergency Department. In particular, we wanted to evaluate whether a new child protection policy for which all staff were trained was being implemented at the local level. The project raised a number of important issues concerning policy research in sensitive areas. An Emergency Department in a Western hospital is characteristically a site imbued with medical discourse which constructs particular knowledges about health, illness and patients. Power relations are defined by a hierarchical structure in which doctors are at the top and in which nurses fulfil their orders. Relations with the public who access the service are also prescribed, with health workers holding expert knowledge to which the public need access because of injury or illness.

Children presenting in this situation are susceptible to both positive and negative influences of the expert power held by health staff, and their power as adults. A strict biomedical model tends to see patients as a series of symptoms that need to be treated and often fails to approach the presenting person from a holistic perspective, which includes consulting them about their illness or injury and involving them in a treatment plan (Willis, 1989, 1994). Children may have even more difficulty in this regard than adults, as they are often seen as extensions of their parents rather than individuals in their own right. This contention is supported by the current research, which revealed that if children's views were sought health staff did not indicate it in either the assessment or treatment plans entered in the medical notes, except in a minority of cases. This omission occurred despite research findings of the last ten years clearly indicating that children as young as three can and should be consulted about their own lives (Baumann, 1997; Kendall, 1997). Failing to locate or to make note of the child's views constructs children and young people as passive objects who have no say in explaining what has happened to them or in participating in the treatment that follows. This study further revealed that staff seldom asked children what brought them to the hospital; they also failed to 'read' the injuries inscribed on the child's body as possible abuse or at least as requiring further exploration. The power relations that existed between the child and health worker were loaded in favour of the health worker: the assessment and treatment of the child were in their hands.

In exposing the impact of these power relations, the project exposed the ethics of the health workers. Staff were bound by legal requirements concerning mandatory notification of the suspicion of child abuse and had received training in new policy guidelines, yet they failed to fulfil their responsibilities. How this came about is open to speculation and reflection. Foucault (1984, cited in Rabinow, 1984) suggests that ethical systems are determined by their social contexts, by the sorts of knowledge valid in particular contexts and by relations of power. Therefore, possible interpretations of the failure of the staff to behave ethically in relation to vulnerable children may relate to the medical site where they worked, and the dominance of the biomedical discourse and the power relations that flow from this dominance. Apart from the systemic response there is also the role of the individual to consider, and the deliberate choice to construct oneself as an ethical subject in relation to the self and others (Foucault, 1984, cited in Rabinow, 1984). Therefore, like all of us, health workers face ethical choices. In this situation, however, the workers are a powerful voice in revealing particular beliefs about children and health practices, the existence of child abuse within families, and how they interpret policy that is handed down from above.

Implicit in the new policy was an alternative discourse, which required staff to shift ground from a purely medical model of health care delivery to incorporate a social model of health in which children were to be seen as active participants in their own health. Providing public health care where the Area Health Service is fully government-funded and subcontracts care to private providers reflects a shift to economic rationalist discourses of health care. In practice, this may mean that private health care providers believe they have a choice as to whether they follow State and Area Health Department policy directives. Indeed, contracts between Area Health Services and private providers may allow flexibility in following policy directives that have resource implications. In addition to these structural interconnections of private and public health care, a further factor exists in longstanding work practices, especially for doctors, which emphasize personal autonomy and choice rather than compliance with statutory responsibilities. This research threatened vested interests at a personal and institutional level by scrutinizing the work practices of health workers and critiquing the policy discourses which influenced the medical site that was studied.

Negotiating relationships

A crucial factor in the life of any research drama is the way relationships between all the actors are negotiated at different stages of the research. Negotiation is an ongoing process throughout the life of the project; it includes the composition of the research team, the way in which the 'script' proposals are read by funding bodies and ethics committees, the relations among members of the research team, and the reactions and relations with other actors within the site being investigated. If we accept the proposition that power relations are embedded in all aspects of the research process, the question is raised: how does power change in the context of different relationships? (Pearce, 1993, p. 26). In different acts throughout the play some players took centre stage while others moved out of focus. Actors brought with them their expectations about the project, their experience of research and their views about the process of research relationships. In this drama, the dynamic nature of power relations was evident as the whole cast worked through the scenes of the project. Relationships between research team members and negotiation with a gatekeeper to the research site are two areas where the fluid nature of power relations was evident.

Relationships between team members

At the beginning of the play, the lead character (or chief investigator) of the drama is required to provide both intellectual and political leadership. She or he is often the person who not only brings together a team of researchers with complementary skills but also directs the production of the script to be submitted to backers for funding. Punch (1994, p. 87) asserts that expectations and roles in team research are rarely examined in the research literature. He suggests that a failure to consider these issues can hinder behaviour in the field and lead to conflict about outcomes. The current research team, formed by me, consisted of a tenured academic with research and policy experience (myself) and two other researchers, Kate and Mary, who were PhD students of mine. This meant there was a prior, institutionally defined relationship between us that to some degree scripted my role as supervisor and their roles as students, creating a particular configuration of power relations. However, our collective biographies indicate a slightly different picture. Both Kate and Mary had extensive experience in child protection work, Kate both in Australia and overseas. We had in fact known each other previously due to our shared work interests. This meant that we were able quickly to address the tasks required, working more as colleagues than in supervisor/student roles. Despite this I was institutionally and ethically responsible for the project, and this produced a particular configuration of power relations between us. Mary and Kate were employed as research assistants, and as a result collected most of the data from the medical files. Data collection was time-consuming and repetitive work, which at times led to frustration. My role was to manage the overall project, to analyse the data and write the final report in consultation with the other team members. This division of labour is not uncommon, particularly in university settings. Regular team meetings were held to discuss the progress of the project. This process worked well for some months but, as Act 8 revealed, tensions emerged when Mary questioned my judgment on who should participate in a feedback session to stakeholders, accusing me of excluding her. At the time it was not clear to me that Kate and Mary, who were friends, had fallen out over an incident outside of the research project. My approach was to explain the reasons behind my decision and to enforce it by reference to my role as chief investigator. This approach suggests that I used the professional power of my roles (as chief investigator, tenured academic and expert in the field) to achieve what I thought was agreement. At the time I felt I had dealt with the issue. However, on reflection it seems to me that relationships within the three-member team deteriorated from that point. This suggests that I missed a critical moment in the research process to manage the manifestations of power within the team relationship. While in this instance the conflict did not hinder the successful completion of the project, relationships were harmed by our collective failure to adequately address the tensions. There is a need to reflect on the characteristics of co-researchers, such as gender, age, experience, prior relationships, status and personality, as potential team members, and to consider conflict resolution strategies at the time of forming a research team.

Relationship with gatekeepers

Access to the field or site where research is to be conducted is a primary focus of researchers; gatekeepers such as the District Health Manager were crucial to the project being able to proceed. In relation to this project the District requested and actively lobbied for the study to be carried out in their area as opposed to other sites we were considering. The reasons for this are unclear; possibly some kudos was perceived from having university research carried out in the hospital. Agreement to participate was therefore more willingly given than in many situations where researchers must convince the gatekeepers of a site or participants to be involved. A meeting was held where we worked out access arrangements, and explored Ethics

Committee clearance and time frames. A formal memo was produced and circulated to the District Manager and me by Kate, who, apart from working as a research assistant on the project, held an Area managerial role. Formally this is more than adequate. However, it has been suggested that 'people who agree to have social scientists study them have not had the experience before and do not know what to expect, nor are they aware of the experience of others social scientists have studied' (Becker, 1964, cited in Denzin, 1989, p. 260). This circumstance raises a number of ethical concerns, which at the time were not clear.

Should I have done as Denzin (1989) suggests and warned the District Manager of the possibility of negative findings and prepare him for the possible consequences? Is this strategic at the point of negotiating access to the site? While formal Ethics Committee procedures stress the need to do no harm, they tend to focus on individual participants in research rather than on organizations. At the time I believed that if the organization was willing to be involved then it would have foreseen the possibility of negative results. This position assumes a shared understanding of research processes and outcomes, which subsequent events revealed to be unfounded. The experience of this project suggests that negotiating access to the site needs to include a discussion of possible outcomes for the organization. Although this may jeopardize access in some settings, not to do so seems less than ethical and positions the researcher as withholding knowledge and running the risk of 'spoiling the field' for other researchers (Punch, 1994).

The politics of negative findings

The data analysis and writing up of the findings highlights another critical moment in the research drama. My selection of excerpts from the final report outlined in Act 7 is clearly subjective. The excerpts highlight for me crucial points within the final fifty-page report, revealing the hidden reality of children's experiences in accessing an Emergency Health Service and telling a story of health system failure despite policy change and extensive training of staff. As Kincheloe and McLaren (1998, p. 260) observe:

> ... *qualitative research that frames its purpose in the context of critical theoretical concerns still produces, in our view, undeniably dangerous knowledge, the kind of information and insight that upsets institutions and threatens to overturn sovereign regimes of truth.*

By interrogating health practices at a local level, existing knowledge and power relations within the organization were challenged; an alternative, dangerous knowledge about the Health Service was presented. No health service wants it known that it fails to care adequately for children and their families who use its services.

The preparation of the report and its subsequent 'opening night' performance for the stakeholders (Act 9) highlights what happens when the research findings reflect badly on individuals, a group or an organization. Mr Grey, as Manager of the Health Service where the research took place, attempted through a number of actions to challenge the knowledge obtained by the research. The Health Area circulated a copy of the report two days prior to a meeting scheduled to discuss the findings. It appears Mr Grey was attempting to reconfigure the power relations inherent in the research process by failing to attend the stakeholder opening night and sending a more junior member of staff. He disputed the methodology, though he was never able to articulate what he thought was invalid. Becker (1970, cited in Herdman, 2000, p. 696) argues that, regardless of the institution studied, the resulting report will anger some people. He argues that the relationship between a social scientist and those studied often contains elements of irreducible conflict, because organizations and communities are internally differentiated and the interests of subgroups differ. The research findings indicated that the service for which Mr Grey was responsible was failing to meet its legal and moral responsibilities to vulnerable and at-risk children and their families. Within the bureaucratic structure of the health service, the research team was a relatively uncontrollable element in an otherwise highly controlled system (Lee, 1993, p. 9). Mr Grey's actions suggest he felt the need to reassert control over the issue.

His next response involved a telephone call to me in which I felt he attempted to intimidate me, threatening legal action. This retreat to a coercive form of power relations seemed to arise because Mr Grey was primarily concerned with protecting the reputation of the organization and was fearful of public exposure of the inadequacies of its response to vulnerable children and their families. A failure to meet children's health needs occurred again in the response to the report findings. The focus was on damage control through refuting methodology and threatening legal action about a confidential research report that had limited distribution and was never intended for public distribution. Additional attempts were made by the District Service to undermine the credibility of the research by approaching the Area Health Service and unsuccessfully arguing that another researcher should repeat the study. Another strategy involved a professor in my university who works closely with the Health Service contacting me at home (while I was on study leave) and lobbying me on the District's behalf. A number of political and ethical questions arise for me in reflecting on the actions of Mr Grey and myself. Would he have attempted to intimidate me if I had been a male researcher? Would it have been different if the research were positivist? Would I have handled it differently if he were a woman? What role did the existence of an all-woman research team investigating how children and their families were treated by a male-dominated health system play in the research process? Throughout this project gender issues were not central to the politics of the play, but it seems useful to remember that this form of power relations can influence not only the position of the researcher but also the roles and actions of the other players in the research drama.

As discussed previously, doing research requires us to take sides. This suggests that the likelihood of making someone angry was high (Herdman, 2000). However, on reflecting after the event it is possible there were different ethical ways in which the response to negative findings could have been minimized. For example, establishing a steering committee for the project including representatives from the site may have provided a forum for educating key players about research and preparation for negative findings. This may have avoided the researched being 'left seething with rage and determined to skin alive the next aspiring ethnographer who seeks access' (Punch, 1994, p. 92). However, this strategy may also raise its own ethical dilemmas for researchers, who must be careful not to be seduced by relationships with the researched, or to be reluctant to make negative findings.

The final act?

The funding body, the National Council for the Prevention of Child Abuse, by implication appears to be an advocate for children. By agreeing to fund this study, this body gave us permission to find out what was going on in the field. The research therefore took place within a funding context of advocacy. As described in Act 11, the funding body subsequently refused to publish the report because it was 'too sensitive'. This occurred despite a revision that removed all reference to the District Health Service and individuals. Despite verbal assurances as to the quality of the report and its usefulness as an 'internal departmental reference', it appears the funding body has also chosen sides. The losers in this situation are vulnerable children and their families.

In spite of the invitation throughout this research to succumb to 'a spiral of silence', I have resisted. The Area Health Service has subsequently contracted me to replicate the study in two other districts; when these studies are completed I will prepare an article for publication on the findings of all three sites. I will have to wait till then to see how publishers respond. In the meantime, this presentation of 'dangerous knowledge' and the reflexive and critical analysis of the project is one act of resistance in challenging the silence about how vulnerable children and their families may be ethically abandoned by a health service. I think this case study supports the proposition that research is a highly contested process, and I hope that this reflexive analysis will assist other social researchers to struggle with the political and ethical dilemmas raised in other critical moments of qualitative research.

Acknowledgement
Thanks to Deb Horsfall, 'Kate McFeast' and Louise Shortus for great feedback at critical moments in writing this.

[1]The definition I am using for physical and sexual violence includes all forms of violence between intimates, whether they be adults or children.

References

Baumann, S. L. (1997) Qualitative research with children as participants. *Nursing Science Quarterly*, **10**(2), 68–69.

Carmody, M. (1992) Uniting all women – a historical look at attitudes to rape. In *Crimes of Violence: Australian Responses to Rape and Child Sexual Assault* (J. Breckenridge and M. Carmody, eds), pp. 7–17. Sydney: Allen and Unwin.

Carmody, M. and Carrington, K. (2000) Preventing sexual violence? *Australian and New Zealand Journal of Criminology*, **33**(3), 241–261.

Denzin, N. K. (1989) On the ethics and politics of sociology. In *The Research Act: A Theoretical Introduction to Sociological Methods*, 3rd edn (N. K. Denzin, ed.), pp. 248–268. Englewood Cliffs: Prentice Hall.

Denzin, N. K. (1997) *Interpretive Ethnography: Ethnographic Practices for the 21st Century*. Thousand Oaks: Sage.

Denzin, N. K. and Lincoln, Y. (eds) (1994) *Handbook of Qualitative Research*. Thousand Oaks: Sage.

Garbarino, J. (1995) *Raising Children in a Socially Toxic Environment*. San Francisco: Jossey-Bass.

Gilbert, N. (ed.) (1994) *Researching Social Life*. London: Sage.

Guba, E. G. and Lincoln, Y. S. (1989) *Fourth Generation Evaluation*. Newbury Park: Sage.

Hallett, C. (1993) Co-ordination and child protection, a review of the literature. *Parent and Child Involvement in Decision Making*. Sydney: NSW Child Protection Council.

Helfer, R. E. and Kempe, C. H. (1976) *Child Abuse and Neglect: The Family and the Community*. Cambridge: Balinger.

Herdman, E. (2000) Reflections on 'making someone angry'. *Qualitative Health Research*, **10**(5), 691–702.

James, A. and Prout, A. (1990) A new paradigm for the sociology of childhood? Provenance, promise and problems. In *Constructing and Reconstructing Childhood: Contemporary Issues in the Sociological Study of Childhood*, pp. 7–34. London: The Falmer Press.

Kendall, J. (1997) The use of qualitative methods in the study of wellness in children with attention deficit hyperactivity disorder. *Journal of Child and Adolescent Psychiatric Nursing*, **10**(4), 27–35.

Kincheloe, J. L. and McLaren, P. L. (1998) Rethinking critical theory and qualitative research. In *The Landscape of Qualitative Research: Theories and Issues* (N. K. Denzin and Y. S. Lincoln, eds), pp. 260–299. Thousand Oaks: Sage.

Lee, R. M. (1993) *Doing Research on Sensitive Topics*. London: Sage.

Parton, N., Thorpe, D. and Wattam, C. (1997) *Child Protection, Risk and the Moral Order*. Hampshire: Macmillan Press Ltd.

Pearce, S. (1993) Negotiating. In *Reflecting on Research Practice: Issues in Health and Social Welfare* (P. Shakespeare, D. Atkinson and S. French, eds), pp. 25–35. Buckingham: Open University Press.

Punch, M. (1994) Politics and ethics in qualitative research. In *Handbook of Qualitative Research* (N. K. Denzin and Y. S. Lincoln, eds), pp. 83–97. Thousand Oaks: Sage.

Rabinow, P. (ed.) (1984) *Michel Foucault, Ethics, Subjectivity and Truth, The Essential Works of Michel Foucault, 1954–1984*, Vol. 1. Lawrence, Kansas: The Allen Press.

Rayner, M. (1991) Children's rights in Australia ... do we need 'The Convention'?. *Twelve to Twenty-five*, **1**(3), 22–25.

Reinharz, S. (1992) *Feminist Methods in Social Research*. New York: Oxford University Press.

Shakespeare, P., Atkinson, D. and French, S. (1993) *Reflecting on Research Practice: Issues in Health and Social Welfare*. Buckingham: Open University Press.

Willis, E. (1989) *Medical Dominance*. Sydney: Allen and Unwin.

Willis, E. (1994) *Illness and Social Relations*. Sydney: Allen and Unwin.

15

Crises of representation

Judy Pinn

When there is a crisis of representation we are freed from the intellectual myopia of hyperdetermined research projects and their formulaic write-ups ... We can turn uncertainty to our advantage; we can be more sociologically imaginative in our thinking, apprehending, and writing of the social world. (Richardson, 1997, p. 14)

Recently I was interviewed as part of some imaginative research into creativity being undertaken by Briony,[1] a postgraduate student. She chose to return the interviews to us for verification, not as the literal transcript of the conversation, but in poetry or prose form. I received some prose that was a pure delight to read and exhilarating to contemplate as a representation of my thoughts on creativity. It was as if the interviewer had seen into my world more fully than my words had articulated and she had represented to me an accurate yet embellished story, with which I was delighted, because it gave me new insights into my creative world. I know her other subject was equally inspired by Briony's poetic representation of his thoughts.

She took a risk and was nervous waiting for our responses to her creative transcriptions, but for her it was a necessary step in her critical exploration of qualitative research. This was the first time I had experienced being the subject of research where the researcher was experimenting with forms of representation that she hoped would provide an alive and fluid interpretation of other people's worlds. It added another dimension to my experiences in qualitative research, in relation to representation. I have also supervised a number of students who have devised imaginative forms of representation for their theses, and I have ventured into writing a 'messy' text (Lincoln and Denzin, 1994, p. 577) as a way of representing some difficult research that I undertook. I will be telling some of these stories more fully, later in the chapter.

A crisis of representation is depicted by Lincoln and Denzin (1994) as one of several crises currently facing qualitative research. Interestingly, when I began this chapter I was writing about a 'crisis of confidence'. When I completed it, it was apparent to me and to the editors that I had written about crises of representation. There is a clear link between the two that will come through in this chapter.

Research is a creative process, and as we begin we are soon faced with questions such as: Can I do this? What am I capable of? What do I want to find out? How will I represent my findings? Qualitative research is a messy, alive, risky and uncertain process. While engaging in open-ended processes such as research it is common to have our confidence tested, perhaps even shaken to the point of crisis. At worst, a crisis in confidence in the process of researching can be painful, debilitating and sometimes embarrassing. At best, moments of high stress and crisis may provide a breakthrough, a critical moment of recognition, that may lead to creative new research directions including new forms of representation.

The dominant social story that is perpetuated through most qualitative research representations, such as reports, papers, journal articles and books, is that the research and its writing up was undertaken with ease, that it was a straightforward event with clear outcomes. This representation of research and writing can undermine the confidence of novice researchers whose experience is otherwise (Richardson, 1994). Overlaying this simplified form of representation is a shifting qualitative research culture that is in a borderland between modernism with its certainty and truth about self and the world, and postmodernism with its uncertainty and fragmentation of truth. As researchers we are embedded in this borderland, which Lincoln and Denzin (1994, p. 583) describe as:

> ... a new age where messy, uncertain multivoiced texts, cultural criticism, and new experimental works will become more common, as will more reflexive forms of fieldwork, analysis and intertextual representation.

Negotiating these shifting cultural frameworks, as we do research, necessarily ruffles our confidence. Producing knowledge that can validly illuminate aspects of human endeavour, responsibly exercising the power that comes with creating knowledge, and being ethically vigilant while opening our work to peer examination and public scrutiny, can be daunting at the best of times. Add to this the epistemological confusion and movement that is occurring in our culture, and which we as researchers must negotiate, and it is not surprising that our confidence will be tested.

In the face of this challenge, I focus in this chapter on how we can use this experience of loss of certainty and confidence to open us to new possibilities rather than to despair. These possibilities include 'writing in' our nervousness, our crises and our anxieties, rather than writing them out, as often happens. To counteract the dominant story of the way in which research is undertaken and represented I will tell some stories, both from my perspective as a researcher and as a supervisor of others' research. I have chosen stories because they provide an embodied description of the excitement and struggle of working with uncertainty. Also, through stories, some of the outcomes, in terms of imaginative forms of representation, are more vivid. In the following stories, multiple crises of confidence, representation, voice, self and knowledge intersect in complex ways. In these stories, the crises were transformed into useful, exciting and creative research. This is not always the case.

Oldfather and West (in Burns-McCoy, 1997) describe qualitative research methodologies as being like jazz: they are fluid improvisations, collaborations, ever shifting and interdependent. These fluid interpretations are increasingly being reflected in the ways researchers are choosing to represent their work. Issues of representation occur because, for some of us, there is an ethical need to question critically the social and power relationships that are being reproduced in our representations. Lincoln and Denzin (1994, p. 577) say that the crisis of representation:

> *... asks the questions, Who is the Other? Can we ever hope to speak authentically of the experience of the Other, or an Other? And if not, how do we create a social science that includes the Other? The short answer is that we move to including the Other in the larger research processes that we have developed.*

This chapter treats particularly the ways in which we 'move to including the Other in the larger research processes' from four interlinked perspectives: theorizing difference, finding voice, changing notions of the self, and competing knowledges. The stories I tell show how some researchers have approached some of the questions raised by the crises of representation.

Theorizing difference

> *At this moment when so much controversy is configured around issues of 'difference', we must ask of writers, artists, and all cultural workers, 'From which discrete set of cultural resources does this person construct his or her discourse?'. (Becker, 1996, p. 18)*

Qualitative research is invariably about relationships, about participating with others – research subjects, auspicing institutions, peers, supervisors, other researchers, even families and friends – to produce knowledge. Within this mix of people there will almost certainly be some differences and possible conflicts that as researchers we need to negotiate. Knowing how to do that, knowing the position from which we work with difference, and being able to theorize our position, are important aspects of the crisis of representation. I will start with a story of my own about difference that shook my confidence and resulted in a different kind of research report.

Judy

The research was a funded project that was designed to develop models of education for HIV/AIDS within Sydney's Cambodian and Vietnamese cultural communities. There was huge conflict, much of which was subterranean, between the seven researchers (three female, four male; two Cambodians, two Vietnamese, one Lebanese, and two Anglo-Australians). The research was an action research project based in both a university and a community. As one of the two university team leaders, very early in the research my dominant feeling was to return the money and disappear! Our difficulties began on day one and lasted until the project was well over. It was hurriedly designed, limited by the funding agency's demands, and caught in the tensions, conflicts, assumptions and different expectations within the team and within all of our cultural communities. It was difficult to maintain the momentum, and I frequently felt in crisis, confronted by ethical, cultural and gender issues that I seemed unable to negotiate.

We made mistakes. Despite what seemed to me to be an enormous mess, we nevertheless had some mixed success. The external assessor employed by the funding agency noted that we had been very 'successful' in our action in the Cambodian community, but seemed to have made 'no difference' in the Vietnamese sector. Within the team we also had some shared moments of learning, achievement, laughter and friendship.

The co-leader and I decided to write our research report with as little sanitizing as possible. We noted all the difficulties and mistakes we made, and provided recommendations to the funding agency about what they might do to prevent future difficulties. Because of the conflict we felt we could not adequately write on behalf of the other researchers, and so we included unedited reports from each of them, an example of Lincoln and Denzin's (1994, p. 577) 'messy' text, 'where multiple voices speak ... often in conflict, and where the reader is left to sort out which experiences speak to his or her personal life'. Some of the things written by one team member felt very unfair to me, and did not represent my experience of the situation at all. Ironically, as co-leader of the research, and holding a certain amount of institutional power, I experienced being represented as 'Other', the one being spoken about! This document sits as a reminder to me that misunderstandings and conflict can happen, and I now acknowledge that at the time we dealt with it as ethically as we could.

This research occurred ten years ago. In reconstructing the experience, I think that my faltering confidence was to a large extent due to feeling out of control of something that was extremely complex. My (gendered?) ethical concern to 'make everything all right for everybody', and my fear that I would say or do inappropriate things, silenced me to some extent and contributed to my being unable to deal effectively with this conflicted situation. Also, I lacked a theoretical framework for dealing adequately with such complexity. We were a group with very different knowledges, ways of knowing and experiences, so clearly we were going to have differences. Most of those differences involved issues of power, and the nature of those power issues changed with particular circumstances. For example, there were power differences between us and the funding agency, and between the university researchers and the community researchers, and there were gender and cultural differences within the group and within the wider community in which we were working. These issues of knowledge, power and authority were complex and, for any understanding to develop within the research group, we needed time to strengthen our relationships through conversations, explore the relevant theory and to live through and understand the conflict we were experiencing. It was time that we didn't have.

I now have an evolving theoretical position that is helping me to re-story this research. We stumbled on the idea of writing the research report in the way we did; we had not heard of 'messy' texts. If I had had access to adequately theorized ideas about this kind of research then, or the confidence to theorize our mess myself, it would certainly have eased some of the pain that I felt while undertaking it. Hooks (1994, p. 59) writes:

> *I came to theory because I was hurting ... I came to theory desperate, wanting to comprehend – to grasp what was happening around and within me. Most importantly, I wanted to make the hurt go away. I saw in theory then a location for healing.*

Theory has also been healing for me. And as Richardson (1997, p. 49) reminds me, theoretical stances are indicative of the subjective state of theorists and of their concern and interest in human agency, power relationships and social order. For example, the intersection of critical, feminist, poststructuralist theory with theories of creativity and imagination is helping me to work more effectively with different knowledges (situated knowledge, partial knowledge and subjugated knowledge), and to be more aware of the politics of difference. As well, these theoretical approaches enable me to provide a space for myself and my students to experiment with ways of representing those knowledges through, for example, the 'messy text' approach to writing 'self' and 'other' (Fine, 1994; Lincoln and Denzin, 1994) and the use of metaphoric, poetic, artistic and performative work (Richardson, 1994, 1997; Mienczakowski, 1997; Heck, 1998). By restor(y)-ing my personal struggle as a woman in relation to working with difference my interest has been sparked in this area, and my current research is directly about working with difference, and imaginative representations of difference, in community.

Reflecting on experiences and theorizing them (preferably as you go) is an essential part of dealing with issues of confidence. Each crisis and experience of dissonance usually represents an important critical moment in the research, and often they are not isolated experiences that you are having alone. Because these are often hidden, even denied, and not included in any reporting of the research, development of exploratory and enabling theories relating to such crises have been hampered.

Finding voice

> ... for it is not difference which immobilises us, but silence. And there are so many silences to be broken. (Lorde, 1984, p. 44)

> ... many social scientists now recognise that no picture is ever complete, that what is needed is many perspectives, many voices, before we can achieve deep understandings of social phenomena, and before we can assert that a narrative is complete. (Lincoln and Denzin, 1994, p. 580)

For many of us, qualitative research and its attendant crises of representation are both about *finding our own voice* and *representing the voices of others*. In a way, finding our own voice through research is a quest for confidence. Both of these intentions are fraught with ontological, epistemological and ethical dilemmas (Fine, 1994). As a supervisor, I have seen students falter and then resolve these dilemmas in methodologically creative ways that, in some instances, also led to challenging the thesis genre. Indeed, the impetus for both the methodology and the subsequent genre challenge came from the researchers' passionate need to have their voices heard. The following two stories are illuminative.

Peter

Peter was a Masters student, who was writing his researching experiences as a story, to get him started in his writing. When it came time to 'switch' into writing in a more conventional academic style, it didn't work for him: he felt that he wasn't expressing what was important for him. He became despondent and considered giving up. So we agreed that he would write the bulk of his thesis as a story. It was a Renaissance story of his collaboration with other artists, including me as his supervisor. Each of us was presented as a character. I, for example, was Sister Judicas; he was Giotto the Renaissance architect. He gave voice to the 'Others' using characters and expressions that felt comfortable to him. The Others were shown his story, and were invited to make comment. The last third of his thesis was written more formally, helped by the preceding story. As often happens in research, his process for finding his voice, his methodology and his way of expressing his research, emerged from the doing, rather than following closely a pre-determined plan. He was later able to find literature that helped him to theorize, name and support the position he had intuitively taken.

The process of writing the story in a way that would be acceptable for a thesis was still difficult, and he experienced both doubt and elation through-out the process of writing. The examiners were both challenged and delighted by his approach, their reports validating the risk he took and adding to his sense of confidence that had arisen through his risk-taking. One of the examiners told me some time later that the thesis had been a kind of watershed for him. He had had to move from his comfortable position as a long-time conventional thesis examiner to a more precarious position, where he had to reconsider the whole process of thesis writing and of exam-ining. What I appreciated about both examiners' comments was their will-ingness to share their vulnerability in the examining process:

> ... when I first discovered that this thesis was partly based on a series of ongoing conversations with key persons or characters, I did wonder at first about the academic appropriateness of this kind of, let us say, 'casual knowl-edge' ... It is a very big challenge to conventions and entrenched habits, and it is a challenge that fully succeeds, I believe, in the special task of redrawing and recreating the world of knowledge. (Examiner 1)

> More conventional theses are easier to examine. The criteria of excellence are well established and the reader can anticipate a certain sequentiality of evi-dence, argument and conclusion. The present study has to be taken as a whole, as evidence, argument and conclusion are not analysed separately. The abstract argument is embedded in the narrative and the information can-not be separated from the process of acquiring the information. It is a difficult task well executed. (Examiner 2)

My confidence as a supervisor was also tested, as I learned to walk a thin line between being supportive of Peter's processes and guiding him regard-ing certain academic conventions that I believed needed to be followed.

Of course, finding one's voice does not mean that the thesis or research has to be 'on the edge' to this extent. However, the process of finding one's voice and representing the voices of others involved in the research is bound to raise issues of confidence. Finding our own voice means not so much discovering a voice that is already there, but consciously fashioning one from the competing stories in which we are embedded.

I encourage students to write about their misgivings, their crises and their personal demons and monsters, by writing their first thoughts about what-ever their issue is – for example, 'what have I got to say that is important?', 'I can't write', or 'I'm a fraud and it's just a matter of time until I'm found out', or 'how can I speak for others?'. They may or may not choose to use the writing in their final thesis draft or article, but often in problematizing part of the research process, it can become an integral part of the methodology section. As Haber (1994, p. 5) points out, when we share and write about our personal fears and our 'deviant' behaviours, we discover that they are not some 'monstrous, idiosyncratic aberration'. When we take these personal experiences into the public realm, not only does it help us to find our voice, we also add to the collective understanding of the research process and enable the politicizing of marginalized voices. Neruda (in Tarn, 1975, p. 217) speaks of the power of this kind of writing in an excerpt from his poem 'Poetry':

> *I did not know what to say, my mouth*
> *had no way*
> *with names,*
> *my eyes were blind,*
> *and something started in my soul,*
> *fever or forgotten wings,*
> *and I made my own way,*
> *deciphering that fire,*
> *and I wrote the first faint line,*
> *faint, without substance, pure nonsense,*
> *pure wisdom,*
> *of someone who knows nothing,*
> *and suddenly I saw*
> *the heavens*
> *unfastened and open,*
> *planets, palpitating plantations,*
> *shadow perforated*
> *riddled*
> *with arrows, fire and flowers,*
> *the winding night, the universe.*

Probably more difficult than finding one's own voice, and for me more ethically fraught, is representing the voices of Others in their multiplicity. The following story illustrates this.

Kieran

Kieran was a Masters student who resolved her ethical dilemma of how to represent the multiple voices of the Others in her research by writing her thesis in four voices. Each represented a different aspect of her role as a researcher: the theorizer/conceptualizer, who theorized the research; the conceptualizer/reflector, who offered critique; the participant/observer, who was the narrator holding the disparate parts of the research together; and the participants, who were the individual participant voices from her collaborative research group. Each of these voices was written in a different typeface and placed in a different position on the page. It was a difficult process; however, it resolved the ethical tensions she had in writing a single-voiced monologue. When I checked this story with Kieran, she reminded me that another of her intentions was to subvert the ways theses are written; explicitly to challenge the usual representations.

The issue of how to represent both our own voice and the voices of the subjects of our research often leads to a crisis of confidence and to uncertainty. How do I find my voice? How can/do I represent Others who are involved in my research? When can I speak on behalf of another? When can I not? These issues are at the centre of much of the current qualitative research literature (see, for example, Denzin and Lincoln, 1994).

Changing notions of the self

> *Researcher/writers self-consciously carry no voice, body, race, class, or gender and no interests into their texts. Narrators seek to shelter themselves in the text, as if they were transparent. (Fine, 1994, p. 74)*

As author of your research, you are entering the contested arena of the role of *authority*. Modernism offers us authority in meta-narratives, stable truths and disciplinary experts, and so the author is not in dispute (indeed frequently not even visible in the text). Postmodernism offers us an unsettling of authority in multiple and competing narratives, multiple truths, and local, contextual knowledges (where the author is reflexive and visible). With this movement between positivist ideas of the researcher as being outside the research (the objective, neutral, reporting observer), and the post-positivist notion of the researcher as integrally participating in and affecting the outcomes of the research, we are dealing with *changing notions of the self*, which then become an integral part of the context of researching and how that research will be represented.

Rushdie (1991, p. 88) writes about this challenge to the notion of self and author-ity (and for him it has been a matter of life and death!):

> *... a rigid blinkered absolutist world view is the easiest to keep hold of, whereas the fluid, uncertain metamorphic picture I've always carried around is rather more vulnerable. Yet I must cling with all my might to my own soul; must hold on to its mischievous, iconoclastic, out-of-step clown instincts, no matter how great the storm. And if that plunges me into contradiction and paradox so be it; I've lived in that messy ocean all my life.*

Following is the story of one woman's struggle for a confident, scholastic, and soulful voice – research that was a striving for a creative self that had to be creatively represented – that picks up on Rushdie's ideas.

Annabelle

While undertaking her Masters thesis, Annabelle decided that her way of representing her research interests was to investigate her subject through quilting. She developed nine artquilts, which became 50 per cent of her thesis (the university had to change its rules *en route* to accommodate her approach, as it was the first time someone in the social sciences had argued for it). During the several years of her research, she was often consumed with a lack of desire to be 'academic', frequently wanting to pull out of the programme. Meanwhile, she was producing artquilts with great confidence and success. She also completed an excellent accompanying documentation of the artquilts, but was still having huge doubts about her ability to complete the thesis (only a section covering her theoretical underpinnings and research methodology needed to be done). I had the examiners in place and the exhibition of the quilts was about to open ... and still no final section! Writing full-time over the next six weeks (with full support from me and a looming deadline) she was able to mobilize her desire, and at the same time accommodate the belief she'd held about 'academic' writing that had niggled at her throughout her research, by writing a coherent piece, which she presented in four 'blocks' of writing with a fifth section as a border, mimicking the quilting process and reflecting the thinking she'd been demonstrating throughout her thesis. Part of what was vital to Annabelle was that the exhibition had to be seen, not represented pictorially. The materiality of the artquilts represented Annabelle's embodied process of recreating reality for the viewer; they were a central part of her thesis.

The examiners' comments were highly supportive of the stand Annabelle had taken, and her risk-taking processes were validated. A comment from each of the examiners highlights some of the issues involved in challenging the conventional thesis genre.

> *[Her] decision to eschew a more traditional style of thesis is a brave one, and one which requires both rigorous intellectual work and a willingness to expose her own life, ideas and talents. This she achieves while avoiding self-indulgence. This style of thesis also requires more work of the candidate than the traditional thesis. [She] had not only to familiarize herself with the ideas of others to test them for their relevance, but then to harmonize them and work them into a new creative synthesis in the artquilts. This she has achieved with considerable elegance. (Examiner 1)*

> *... the candidate constructed a methodology both reflexive and reflective, which allowed her to share her strength on her own terms and made a convincing contribution to her area. (Examiner 2)*

Annabelle is now undertaking a PhD, 'on her own terms', with confidence, although I expect it will be punctuated with other critical moments throughout her researching process.

Research undertaken in the social realm is necessarily about 'self' (Krieger 1991). For example, while writing this chapter I asked several people what their research had been about and was told it was 'to understand myself', 'to understand my mother-in-law', 'to reflect on my professional practice', and 'to find my voice', although these insights may have been clearer on reflection than at the start of the research.

Research could be claimed to be about affirming the self as a contradictory, learning, yet fallible human being. However, as I have already mentioned, many researchers get caught in 'feeling fallible', incompetent and inadequate; only one aspect of self. This occurrence has been theorized and called the 'impostor phenomenon', an inner experience of intellectual phoniness, first studied and named in relation to high-achieving women, who despite their achievements persisted in regarding themselves as unintelligent and having fooled those who thought them otherwise. Early family dynamics and later social sex-role stereotyping are major contributing factors to the development of the phenomenon (Clance and Imes, 1978). This phenomenon has also been recognized and researched, in conjunction with issues of fear of failure, fear of success and perfectionism, with African-

American graduate students (Ewing *et al.*, 1996), male and female marketing managers (Fried-Buchalter, 1997), and medical, dental, nursing and pharmacy students (Henning, Ey and Shaw, 1998).

The above studies highlight the need for subjectivity and reflexivity in research. Our processes as researchers, our fears and perfectionism as well as our successes, need to be brought consciously into the research process. In this way we can reveal the uncertainty, contradictions, multiplicities and ambiguities of ourselves. In many ways it is an important ethical stance. Confidence involves accepting that shifting perspective of the self, and then exploring ways of representing it to others.

Competing knowledges

> *Somehow, letting go of the need to have the right answer and adopting a more fluid, less rigid perspective – on anything – allowed an openness to change that felt personally transformative. Since I have begun to see the significance of this approach to knowledge in my own life, it disturbed me that it was not often acknowledged or used ... (Mittman, 1997, p. 4)*

As I was writing this chapter, I went for a walk along an ill-defined path on a cliff edge overlooking the sea. As I walked there were several indications that it was a public path, even though it was very close to the back of people's houses. It petered out and then was well defined again. At one point as I looked ahead the path appeared to end: there was a house built close to the cliff edge and a garden was cultivated where the path should run. I hesitated and for a moment lost my confidence to continue. This appeared to be private land, and if I continued I would be trespassing. Then I realized that there were two competing knowledges at work here: the knowledge that I had been on a public path, and my sudden perception that I might now be on private land. In that critical moment of clashing knowledges I temporarily lost my confidence and was momentarily paralysed. I decided to go ahead, however, and as I walked through the private cultivated garden, right beneath the windows of the house, the public path became apparent again. I surmised that the garden had been built deliberately to create doubt and so stop people walking close to the house.

I tell this story as a metaphor for the relationship between knowledge and confidence. Doubt, brought about by conflicting constructions of stories about how things are, is central to developing understanding and central to research. This doubt, I would say, is my Achilles heel in terms of disturbing my confidence, just as it did on the path. We conduct research because we don't know something and are setting out on a process to find out. This is emotionally and intellectually slippery territory, and frequently we are challenged to unlearn things we hold dear, view the world differently, let sacred cows be slaughtered and live with different ways of knowing and different knowledges. Geertz (1993, p. 234) indicates beautifully at least two of the difficulties this process can raise:

> *... a serious effort to define ourselves among different others ... involves quite serious perils, not least of which are intellectual entropy and moral paralysis.*

Intellectual entropy (I have nothing to say) and moral paralysis (what can I do?) can be precursors to a crisis of confidence and its attendant quandaries about representation. It is often important that we hold knowledge tentatively and lightly. And yet there is such a culture of certainty being reflected back to us. An individual crisis of confidence can easily be triggered when we don't recognize and work with the tension that knowledge is tentative, and that uncertainty and ambiguity are legitimate ways of knowing, while at the same time, for pragmatic reasons, we need to be able to act within this uncertainty.

As researchers, we are expected to claim some *public space*. Indeed, this is one of the prerequisites of research, that our knowledge be made public in a reliable and valid way. In other words, we are necessarily putting our knowledge and the way we constructed it forward for scrutiny, for public comment. It may be in a published refereed work, in a thesis to be judged by examiners, at a conference, to a funding body, or applied back in our organization or community.

Unfortunately there is, in my experience, an academic culture of attack, in relation to different knowledges. This certainly shakes my confidence and frequently encourages me to be conservative in the ways I represent my knowing. At a conference some years ago, a woman academic delivered a paper that she indicated was very tentative and still unfolding in relation to her research area. However, she was keen to obtain some feedback. She was attacked from the audience by several male academics. Following this, a group of women (including myself) who were yet to present our papers spent time both supporting the woman and devising a way in which we could present our work without similarly being attacked. We asked specifically at the beginning of our presentations that others support us with critical discussion, and said that we were unwilling to countenance attack.

Securing this sort of support for your way of knowing, your approach to research and your forms of representation is vital. As a supervisor, I aim to create a space for the researcher to explore her particular ways of knowing. (I have witnessed several researchers lose confidence in their creative endeavours because their supervisor's different way of knowing was 'the only acceptable approach'.) As a researcher, if I feel isolated, I seek people to support me. Often these are other researchers, and our mutually constructed ideas can be included in each of our research documents.

Show me . . . !

> But after so much 'telling' I wanted to 'show'. I used alternative forms of representation: drama, performance pieces, poetry, and finally, alighting on an old form . . . the personal essay, but making it my own, writing both against and within its conventions. (Richardson, 1997, p. 3)

I am aware of the irony in my having written this chapter largely by 'telling' about the crises of representation rather than 'showing' alternative forms of representation. One of my strengths is that I provide a 'container' for others to experiment with different forms of representation, but in doing that I sometimes neglect my own experimentation. I am longing to transgress the forms of representation I have been 'trained' into, and am in the process of doing so in my current research, largely through drama and poetry, because I believe they both have the power to represent the multiplicity of the social world that fascinates me.

Confidence in working with different forms of representation comes from breakthroughs: taking risks and having them pay off; being well supported to push boundaries; being able to write about and theorize our deepest dark secrets about our messy researching process; seeking and receiving useful feedback from supervisors, mentors and peers; recognizing that there is more than one way of knowing, doing and being in the world; and being aware of the cultural and therefore methodological shifts that are currently occurring in the research world.

Research as a creative process, is a story that we tell. Becker (1996, p. 216) encapsulates this creative process well:

> *To be creative one needs to feel the confidence to recreate the world from scratch, to defy order, to break the conventional apart, to analyse and be critical of existing forms, to assert the unconscious over the conscious, to insist on the integration of both. One must make concrete objects into theories of abstract thought and transform abstract thought into the concrete. One must have the confidence to create a personal odyssey and to make one's person the center and subject of the narrative.*

During the research process, a crisis of confidence and a crisis in representation can be reconstructed to our advantage if we consider research to be a practice of uncertainty.

Kincheloe and McLaren (1994, p. 151) speak of this creative and tentative approach as 'research humility', which 'implies a sense of the unpredictability of the sociopolitical microcosm and the capriciousness of the consequences of inquiry'.

Sometimes we present others with a facade of confidence. This can thwart an opportunity to experience the creative resolutions that can sometimes come from the uncertainty about how to represent your understanding of the social world of your research. Confidence is related to being able to rely on our lived experience, to theorize it, and where necessary to transform it in a way that indicates our comfort with fluidity, movement and uncertainty and a willingness to expose ourselves as vulnerable, humble researchers, rather than see ourselves as impostors.

As Kappeler (in Lather, 1991, p. 159) so aptly puts it, I don't want to 'conclude and sum up, rounding off the argument so as to dump it in a nutshell on the reader'. There is always more that could be said, and my hope too is that this chapter is not about 'a set of answers, but making possible a different practice'.

Having said that, the only fitting way that I can finish is 'to show', with a poem of my own struggle with representation, called *I could not settle*:

> *As I sat at my desk to read and write*
> *enamoured as I am of worthy ideas*
> *I could not settle.*
> *I could not settle!*
> *Out into the autumn garden,*
> *dim torch to lead the way*

I picked some early freesias – such fragrance!
And set them on my desk.

But still I could not settle.
I could not settle!
A glass of champagne – such indulgence!
I don't drink champagne so often any more,
and some chocolate gems – such folly!
But sweet with promise of immediate pleasure.
And I set them on my desk.

So now I was ready to begin my scholarly work
but I could not settle
I could not settle!
So I wrote this poem – such joy!
Unfolding, with its own desperate need
for life, for fragrance, for folly and joy
to punctuate those desolate words that
are so respectable and erudite
and that murder me
and cripple the Other.

And I could settle
I could settle.

(3 June 1999)

Acknowledgment
I would like to thank Briony Edwards, Peter Hedley, Kieran Davis and Annabelle Solomon for their willingness to explore the 'edge' in their research, to share their stories, and for the learning we have done together.

[1]All the stories that are told in this chapter have been checked out with the people involved.

References

Becker, C. (1996) *Zones of Contention: Essays on Art, Institutions, Gender, and Anxiety*. Albany: State University of New York Press.

Burns-McCoy, N. (1997) Water is to chocolate like story is to qualitative research: questioning credibility and narrative studies. *The Journal of Critical Pedagogy*, hhtp://www.lib.wmc.edu/pub/jcp/issue1-2/burns-mccoy.html

Clance, P. and Imes, S. (1978) The impostor phenomenon in high achieving women: Dynamics and therapeutic intervention. *Psychotherapy: Theory, Research and Practice*, **15**(3), 241–247.

Denzin, N. and Lincoln, Y. (eds) (1994) *Handbook of Qualitative Research*. Thousand Oaks: Sage.

Ewing, K., Richardson, T., James-Myers, L. and Russell, R. (1996) The relationship between racial identity attitudes, worldview, and African American graduate students' experience of the impostor phenomenon. *Journal of Black Psychology*, **22**(1), 53–66.

Fine, M. (1994) Working the hyphens: reinventing self and other in qualitative research. In *Handbook of Qualitative Research* (N. Denzin and Y. Lincoln, eds), pp. 70–82. Thousand Oaks: Sage.

Fried-Buchalter, S. (1997) Fear of success, fear of failure, and the impostor phenomenon among male and female marketing managers. *Sex Roles*, **37**(11–12), 847–859.

Geertz, C. (1993) *Local Knowledge*. London: Fontana Press.

Haber, H. (1994) *Beyond Postmodern Politics*. New York: Routledge.

Heck, M. (1998) Artmaking and aesthetic inquiry: critical connections among centering, social transformation, and pedagogy. *The Journal of Critical Pedagogy*, hhtp://www.lib.wmc.edu/pub/jcp/issueII-1/heck.html

Henning, K., Ey, S. and Shaw, D. (1998) Perfectionism, the impostor phenomenon and psychological adjustment in medical, dental, nursing and pharmacy students. *Medical Education*, **32**(5), 456–464.

hooks, b. (1994) *Teaching to Transgress. Education as the Practice of Freedom*. New York: Routledge.

Kincheloe, J. and McLaren, P. (1994) Rethinking critical theory and qualitative research. In *Handbook of Qualitative Research* (N. Denzin and Y. Lincoln, eds), pp. 138–157. Thousand Oaks: Sage.

Krieger, S. (1991) *Social Science and the Self*. New Brunswick: Rutgers University Press.

Lather, P. (1991) *Getting Smart: Feminist Research and Pedagogy with/in the Postmodern*. London: Routledge.

Lincoln, Y. and Denzin, N. (1994) The fifth moment. In *Handbook of Qualitative Research* (N. Denzin and Y. Lincoln, eds), pp. 575–586. Thousand Oaks: Sage.

Lorde, A. (1984) *Sister Outsider: Essays and Speeches*. New York: Crossing Press.

Mienczakowski, J. (1997) Theatre of change. *Research in Drama Education*, **2**(2), 159–172.

Mittman, J. (1997) Crossing the borders of critical pedagogy and creative process: a rationale and practical application using improvisational theatre and interactive television with semi-rural teenagers. *The Journal of Critical Pedagogy*, http://www.lib.wmc.edu/pub/jcp/issue1/mittman.html

Richardson, L. (1994) Writing: a method of inquiry. In *Handbook of Qualitative Research* (N. Denzin and Y. Lincoln, eds), pp. 516–529. Thousand Oaks: Sage.

Richardson, L. (1997) *Fields of Play: Constructing an Academic Life*. New Brunswick: Rutgers University Press.

Rushdie, S. (1991) *Midnight's Children*. New York: Penguin.

Tarn, N. (ed.) (1975) *Pablo Neruda: Selected Poems*. Harmondsworth: Penguin Books.

16

Perspectives and dilemmas in thesis examination

Joy Higgs

The term *critical moment* has several meanings in relation to the examination of theses. A *moment* can refer to a point in time, to the moment or importance of an event or idea, and to 'the measure of a force by its power to cause rotation' (Hayward and Sparkes, 1982, p. 742). *Critical* can refer to criticism, to something that is important or essential, and to the act of critiquing. The examination of theses is all of these things. At a point in time the thesis is judged, to assess its worth or importance against essential criteria (e.g. the requirement of a PhD to make a unique contribution to the body of knowledge of the field). In addition, the thesis is assessed against a set of more invisible criteria or yardsticks, known consciously or unconsciously to the examiner who may be swayed by the force and credibility of the argument and the elegant simplicity or scholarship of the presentation or product, or who may 'turn critic' in the absence of substance or quality of writing.

The time of thesis examination is a critical moment for many people: the candidate, the supervisor(s), the many others who have supported and paid the cost of the candidate's toil and turmoil, the school anticipating another successful graduate, and the examiner. With all these critical moments coming together at the end of the candidature, this is an appropriate final chapter in this book, even though for each of these players the question of 'what next?' already hovers in the background while the examination process is being completed.

This chapter is written from the perspective of the examiner. Interestingly, if it were a chapter in a book on empirico-analytical or quantitative research then perhaps it could be reduced to a concise outline of guidelines providing clear standards relating to research performance (objectivity, reliability and validity), and known and well-publicised research strategies. These guidelines would be supported by generations of theses as role models or precedents, and disciplinary traditions in terms of expectations of postgraduate theses.

The role of thesis examiner in the qualitative research arena is more broad and problematic. A number of the dilemmas or critical moments, in all senses of the term, face the qualitative researcher as examiner.

Dilemma 1: Someone chose me as examiner – am I the right person for the job?

> *Dear ... ,*
> *The University of ... has asked me to invite you to be an examiner of a qualitative research thesis titled 'An investigation of nurse–patient interactions in intensive care units'. Please find attached the thesis abstract. Please advise if you would be available to examine this thesis.*

Perhaps, on receiving such a letter, you face a decision rather than a dilemma. You have the time and you feel competent to examine this topic or method. However, there are a number of issues to be addressed that could, indeed, turn this request into a dilemma.

The thesis methodology is labelled qualitative, but this term may be used loosely with many different meanings. To some people any survey study is qualitative, regardless of the fact that some survey studies result in quantified products, statistical analysis and the testing and 'proving' of hypotheses. In essence, such research belongs to the empirico-analytical research paradigm (see Table 16.1).

Table 16.1 The empirico-analytical, interpretive and critical research paradigms (Based on Higgs 1998)

Research paradigm	Research goals	Research approach(es)
Empirico-analytical paradigm	To measure, test hypotheses, discover, predict, explain, control, generalize, identify cause-effect relationships	Experimental method (The scientific method)
Interpretive paradigm	To understand, interpret, seek meaning, describe, illuminate, theorize	Hermeneutics, phenomenology narrative inquiry, naturalistic inquiry
Critical paradigm	To improve, empower, change reality or circumstances	Action research/collaborative research Collaborative and planned action to achieve agreed goals Praxis – acting on existing conditions to change them
Combined paradigms	Mixture of the above	Mixture of the above

While a simple definition of qualitative research is *research that relies on qualitative (non-mathematical) judgments*, the terms quantitative and qualitative research are not ideal. In both cases, qualitative and value-laden judgments can be used and interpretations are made of observations and findings. Similarly, qualitative researchers can use quantitative techniques to analyse data (Higgs and Cant, 1998). To alleviate this terminology concern, researchers could categorize research as belonging to the empirico-analytical, interpretive or critical research paradigms, as outlined in Table 16.1 (and discussed in more detail in Chapter 4).

For the potential examiner, then, it is necessary to look beyond the label 'qualitative' to identify the actual research approach (e.g. by reading the abstract that is provided or obtained). The issue the examiner is confronting is authenticity. That is, the examiner needs to face the task of examining with credibility and with a clear intention of doing justice to judging the research product, which represents extensive endeavour by the candidate.

This issue of authenticity also needs to be addressed in seeking to answer the questions: *Do I know enough about the topic to be a credible examiner? Am I sufficiently knowledgeable of the research method to complete this task responsibly?* With the vast array of research methods falling under the broad qualitative umbrella, it would be a rare examiner who feels equally competent to review research from the traditions of ethnography, phenomenology, hermeneutics, narrative inquiry, phenomenography and action research, for example. The examiner can make neither too much nor too little of this decision.

The examiner's role is to certify the thesis as satisfactory according to the stated and unstated criteria for the degree. The unstated or understood criteria include value judgments of the uniqueness of the research. PhDs, for instance, should make a significant contribution to expanding the knowledge of the selected field. *Can I make this judgment? Do I have relevant and sufficient knowledge?* The examiner must make a judgment on the quality of the research. *What should we expect of an Honours, Masters, PhD or professional doctorate thesis? What yardsticks should I use?* This question is of particular concern to new examiners. Experience in supervision and examining brings practical knowledge to clarify this expectation. Dilemma 4 further explores this matter.

Apart from the tacit or ephemeral or discipline-specific expectations of a thesis, examiners can be asked to address specific judgment criteria. Consider the following instructions to examiners. In agreeing to examine, we are saying that we can appropriately address these criteria. Examiners may need to seek peer assistance, gain experience or pursue professional development to perform this task well.

The university asks examiners to record whether in the opinion of the examiner:

1. *the thesis is a substantially original contribution to the knowledge of the subject concerned*
2. *the thesis affords evidence of originality by the discovery of new facts*
3. *the thesis affords evidence of originality by the exercising of independent critical ability*
4. *the thesis is satisfactory as regards literary presentation*
5. *the research method is appropriate to the topic, and*
6. *a substantial amount of material in the thesis is suitable for publication.*

In relation to the credibility/responsibility issue, it is important to acknowledge that some examiners are chosen on the basis of content expertise, others on methodological grounds and others on both counts. In relation to (1) or (2), a prospective examiner who considers him/herself to be insufficiently knowledgeable to examine all thesis dimensions would need to seek peer assistance in order to make credible comment on thesis content and method, or should decline to be an examiner.

Dilemma 2: Accepting the commission – can I do justice to the research approach and product?

One of the most irksome difficulties facing qualitative researchers is the frequent use of quantitative/experimental research headings and structure as the norm or requirement for theses. Students may be required to follow a traditional quantitative thesis structure such as:

- *Title*
- *Abstract*
- *Acknowledgments*
- *Introduction*
- *Literature review*
- *Aims of the study*
- *Methodology*
- *Analysis*
- *Findings*
- *Discussion of findings*
- *Conclusions*
- *Applications and limitations*
- *References*
- *Appendices. (Burnard, 1992)*

From the examiner's point of view, you may be required to comment on a thesis which is presented in this structure.

Whether or not the student has been required to constrain the thesis into these prescribed headings, examiners (like journal reviewers) often have to produce a report which artificially comments on dimensions or sections not present or desirable in many forms of qualitative theses. Examples of headings used in (liberated) qualitative theses are provided in Table 16.2.

For the student and examiner alike, allowing the structure to match and do justice to the research approach is by far the preferable option.

Dilemma 3: Defining my responsibilities – am I supervisor, editor, critic, expert, evaluator?

What level of decision-making and comment is required of the examiner? One thing is clear: the examiner is required to make a judgment of the standard of the thesis. The form of decision may include a set of options like those contained in Table 16.2. This decision is challenging in that it requires the examiner to have an internal yardstick of what is 'good enough', what is excellent (etc.). The decision is even more difficult if a mark needs to be assigned (see Table 16.3). The instructions assist in differentiating grades, but it is left to the examiner's experience to make the judgment call and differentiate adequate from inadequate. To illustrate this point consider the following story.

Recently, two examiners read the same Honours (undergraduate) thesis. An experienced qualitative researcher who had examined four Doctoral and two Masters theses in the preceding twelve months awarded a mark of 90 to the Honours thesis. The second examiner, a Masters graduate whose main experience was in examining postgraduate coursework treatises (essays)

Table 16.2 Examples of headings used in qualitative research theses

Prototype	*Titchen (2000)*	*Bridgman (2000)*	*Denshire (2000)*	*McCormack (1998)*
Introduction goals, structure Theoretical framework Research approach Philosophical framework Research paradigm Research approach Data collection methods Data analysis methods Strategies to ensure quality of research Ethics approval Research findings/Discussion I (e.g. Participants' narratives) Research findings/Discussion II (e.g. Theoretical model) Critique of research Conclusion References Appendices	• Introductory overview • Approaches to the study of nurses' practical thinking and expertise • Critical review of the substantive literature • The critical social science perspective • Methodology • Skilled companionship: A conceptual framework for patient-centred nursing • Testing the Skilled Companionship framework: Refinement & transferability • Outsider Critical Companionship: A conceptual framework for helping a practitioner to facilitate nurses' acquisition of PCK • Insider Critical Companionship: A conceptual framework for facilitating nurses' acquisition of PCK • Testing the Critical Companionship framework: Refinement and transferability • Conclusions critique and beyond	• Introduction – Re-awakening • Re-formulating – Critique of Science – A Different Storying • Re-working – Women – Identity, Work and Power • Re-searching – Re-search Methodology and Methods – The Storying • Re-flecting – The Process – Singing up the Stories • Re-generating – Creating a Space for a New Mythology • Re-cycling – The Rise and Fall of Women in the Cycles of Her-Story • Re-membering – Women in the Her-story of Medicine • Re-cognising – Women in Medicine Today • Re-creating – Role Models for Women – Re-creating a New Story • Re-balancing – Concluding • Re-stor(y)ing • Re-sources – Bibliography • Appendices	• Exploring the personal and professional • Study design and execution • Findings for metaphor analysis • Findings for terminology-based analysis • Developing a model of reflective practice • Reflections and recommendations	• Introduction • Autonomy – A health care perspective • Philosophical foundations • 'Seeing' autonomy in practice – The search for a methodology • Communicative style • Power and control • 'Speaking for you or speaking for me' • Context, expertise and identified principles for action • Autonomy as authentic consciousness • The nurse as facilitator of authentic consciousness • Limitations, implications and aspirations

Table 16.3 Grading honours theses

Class I (80–100)	Class II, Division 1 (75–79)	Class III, Division II (70–74)
Excellent standard	High standard	Good standard
• Comprehensive review of relevant literature, with evidence of thorough knowledge of relevant theoretical issues	As for Class 1, but the standard is not consistent across all categories	• Review of relevant literature, based on key articles and/or texts, with satisfactory knowledge of relevant theory
• Background information is well integrated and organised		• Background information is not well integrated nor presented
• Demonstrates the relevance of the literature to the proposed study		• Shows some ability to evaluate and analyse evidence
• Demonstrates the ability to analyse and evaluate evidence and arguments at high levels		• Design of the study and methodology procedures correct with some understanding of the strengths and weaknesses of the selected methodology
• Design of the study and methodological procedures correct with the strengths and weaknesses of chosen methodology clearly identified		• Results clearly and correctly presented
• Results clearly and correctly presented		• Statistical analyses have been correctly chosen and interpreted
• Statistical analyses have been correctly chosen and interpreted		• Results are discussed superficially in terms of theory (existing or new), the contribution of the findings to scientific theory or clinical practice; and the potential of the findings to stimulate further research, and
• Results are discussed in terms of theory (existing or new), the contribution of the findings to scientific theory or clinical practice, and the potential of the findings to stimulate further research, and		• Demonstrates clarity of writing style, but with poor overall organisation
• Demonstrates clarity of writing style, material well organised and visual information well presented		

Class III (65–69)	Below 65
Satisfactory standard As with Class II, Division 2, however: • Review of relevant literature limited, with little theoretical knowledge demonstrated • Relevant literature is not integrated and is poorly presented • Design of the study and methodological procedures correct with limited understanding of the strengths and weaknesses of the selected methodology • Results correctly presented although statistical analyses may have been incorrectly chosen and/or interpreted • Superficial discussion of findings, with failure to note how findings contribute to the knowledge base or how they might stimulate further researcher, or • Poor overall organisation of material, poor referencing	Fail/Unsatisfactory Did not achieve the minimal criteria identified for a Class III Honours Award, for example: • Demonstrated a lack of understanding of the theoretical knowledge • Inappropriate or seriously flawed methodology chosen • Demonstrated a lack of competence in presenting the results or in understanding and interpreting the analyses; or • Demonstrated a failure or inability to integrate findings with extant knowledge

(Source: School of Physiotherapy, The University of Sydney, Australia)

gave a mark of 78. Without a yardstick which included higher level post-graduate research, she considered the thesis to be 'very good' but avoided the end of the marking scale. The more experienced examiner recognized this work, at Honours level, to be excellent.

Beyond awarding marks, other forms of comment can be even more problematic. For instance, how does the examiner deal with the request to identify required emendations? A wide range of approaches can be taken. Some examiners:

- comment in detail on every small spelling and format error

Isn't this the job of the candidate with oversight by the supervisor?

- make speeches and demonstrate their own knowledge, perhaps in a mistaken demonstration of credibility

The goal is to assess the value of the candidate's work and knowledge, not the examiner's.

- offer useful advice which may (or may not!) be distinguishable from requirements to amend the thesis

If advice is offered by the examiner it needs to be clearly differentiated from recommended or required emendations. The university committee/decision-maker(s) receiving an examiner's report should be in no doubt what the examiner is expecting of the candidate. Also the examiner should recognize that advice might serve (in magnitude or nature) to diminish recommendations of acceptance of the thesis. The words and arguments of the examiner need to be consistent with the decision or grade awarded.

- require minor or major emendations.

While the examiner's role is to identify any emendations considered necessary to meet the required standard, it is not the examiner's role to enhance the quality, style or presentation of the thesis in excess of the necessary standards for award of the degree. This is the supervisor's role with the candidate, prior to submission of the thesis for examination.

Where one examiner's report is self-contradictory, or where two or three examiners' reports represent different judgments, the university decision-makers (e.g. a postgraduate committee) will need to make a decision on whether the thesis meets the prescribed criteria, and specify the emendations required.

Dilemma 4: Identifying criteria for evaluation – what yardsticks should I use?

The literature is replete with discussions of criteria for evaluating qualitative research (Guba and Lincoln, 1994; Leininger, 1994; Goodfellow, 1997; Higgs and Adams, 1997; Thorne, 1997; McAllister, 1998). Within this breadth of opinion and criteria lies the opportunity to set criteria for judging the nature and essence of different forms of qualitative research, as well as a minefield for the novice or unwary. The examiner needs to come to terms with several issues related to the topic of criteria for evaluating qualitative research.

The principal issue is the inappropriateness of adopting quantitative research evaluation criteria blindly in an endeavour to gain credibility for qualitative research in a world dominated by the practice language and standards of quantitative research. Neither is it desirable to simply transform quantitative criteria (validity, reliability, objectivity) and goals (generalizability, rigour) via word changes. Thorne (1997, p. 118) argues that major problems with qualitative research reflect 'epistemological confusion and the inappropriate application of quantitative measures to an entirely distinct epistemological enterprise'.

Traditionally, the positivist paradigm sets four criteria as necessary for quality in its research (Denzin and Lincoln, 1994). These criteria are:

- *internal validity* (the extent to which the research findings correctly portray the phenomenon being investigated)
- *external validity* or generalizability (the extent to which the findings of the study can be generalized to similar settings)
- *reliability* (the extent to which the research findings can be reproduced or replicated by another researcher)
- *objectivity* (the extent to which the research findings are free of bias).

A wide variety of terms are used in qualitative research to describe quality. Several themes emerge within this range of terminology, including the need for:

- *credibility* (the outcomes are reasonable and sound in light of the question posed and method adopted)
- *soundness* (the method has credibility and has been implemented authentically; the method is congruent with the phenomenon being investigated, the context and the research paradigm articulated)
- *ethicality* (the research was conducted ethically with particular reference to participants in the project)
- *quality writing* (including ideas of scholarly writing, and writing that is compatible with the research phenomenon, audience and method, e.g. 'rich and resonant' (in narrative inquiry) (Goodfellow, 1997), 'poetic language' (in phenomenology) (Smith, 1997) and 'language which makes the event or phenomenon and the people involved come alive' (in ethnography) (Fitzgerald, 1997))
- *a valuable contribution* (the research is deemed to have made a substantial contribution, to have provided new insights to knowledge, or to have added to the measure of well-being of human society).

Research that could be considered outstanding would need to exhibit additional features. For instance, it could demonstrate:

- *immortality* (outstanding research bestows a measure of immortality on its artisans through the contribution it makes to knowledge; this could include seminal work, benchmark findings or pivotal changes in patterns of thought or research strategy)

- *power* (powerful research achieves much of the enormous potential available to qualitative research, presenting its findings in a rich and powerful manner (see Morse, 1997))
- *quality as a lived experience and strategy* (in such research there is seamlessness between the person as self, ethical performer and researcher)
- *embodied knowing* (in such research the authenticity of implementation comes from direct acting-out of deeply held positions and values; actions are an extension rather than a practised or crafted adoption of the principles underlying the research philosophy)
- *challenge to self and the system* (such embodied research demonstrates a willingness and adeptness in breaking new boundaries, extending both self and system).

I provide several extracts from thesis examination reports to illustrate such exceptional achievement. These are quoted but not referenced, to protect the anonymity of the writers and candidates.

> *This is an exemplary thesis which makes a major contribution to knowledge in the fields of ...*

Among the strengths listed are:

> *A sophisticated analysis of three major methodological literatures and a generation of a research designed from a skilful synthesis of key aspects of all three. Chapters 4 and 5 which contain this work are a* tour de force.

> *A clear, simple structure for the thesis, which enables the highly complex methodology and conceptualizations to be presented with admirable clarity.* (*Elegant simplicity in action! Immortality*)

> *I am very impressed by the depth and richness of this work; its freshness and harmony of language, mode and message. The candidate realizes with scholarship and soul her intended outcomes. In essence, this work achieves the outcome of being true to self, to the research goals, to the theoretical framework provided and the research approach. This is a very fine achievement.* (*Authenticity and embodiment*)

> *This was a challenging and exciting project. The candidate has taken a unique approach to researching a difficult topic via autobiography. The work is illuminating, insightful and expansive of knowledge in the field. The thesis combines a depth of practice understanding with personal reflection, insightful literature access and creative autobiographical research into the development of a meaningful model of occupational understanding.* (*Challenging*)

In a research project entitled 'An exploration of dimensions of implementing qualitative research', Higgs and Radovich (1999) found that quality in the research process became a lived strategy for experienced and highly competent qualitative researchers. Such researchers demonstrated:

- a deep understanding of the philosophical framework of their research
- a recognition of the value of achieving a high level of congruence between the various dimensions of research design and implementation, including the research structure (i.e. the paradigmatic and theoretical frameworks) and the research process

- a deep knowledge of the theoretical framework of the research project both in preparation for selection or construction of the research question and research design and as a parallel process to the collection and analysis of data
- a willingness to experiment with new research strategies or with research approaches which cross or push forward paradigm boundaries
- adoption of a metacognitive research approach focusing on achievement of quality criteria through continuous self, process and outcome monitoring and process reflection
- a type of embodied research knowing highlighted by vitality, assurance, deep understanding of chosen research strategies, strong sense of self as a researcher and use of metacognitive strategies to achieve planned and espoused objectives or ethical/quality goals
- high levels of personal challenge, reflection, critique, and the courage to change directions and to challenge orthodoxy.

Conclusion

Examiners of qualitative research theses are grown, not born. Through personal experience as research students, supervisors and examiners, through informal learning (e.g. peer consultation and advice) and through professional development (e.g. supervisory training programmes), qualitative researchers learn to deal with the dilemmas of thesis examination and gain the necessary perspectives, standards and expertise to be competent examiners. Many of these issues are also applicable to related tasks such as grant application and journal paper reviewing, where the language and precedence of empirico-analytical research often dominates decision-making and the researcher is expected to compete or gain approval in a context which is not of her or his choosing. Beyond the development needs of individual examiners and reviewers there also need to be system changes that bring new perspectives to theses and thesis examination criteria and requirements, to enable the essence and quality of qualitative research to be better understood, demonstrated and examined.

Two core arguments are presented in this paper:

- To have a vision of how to deal with these critical moments is to understand that research and decisions about research are encapsulated within the character and identity of *cultures*, the understandings and limitations inherent in *language* and the expectations and notions associated with *quality and scholarship*.
- To change the acceptability of qualitative research for examiners, reviewers and other decision-makers requires *education and action*. Qualitative researchers need to understand and change the context in which they are seeking acceptance. This requires education of qualitative researchers in the identification and attainment of quality in research, and education of the decision-makers in terms of broadening (rather than softening) the scope and criteria for judging quality in research. Research managers, such as chairs of ethics and grant committees and committees which set requirements for thesis examination or publications

reviewing, also need to change their approaches. Criteria and guidelines for thesis submission and research proposals need to encompass the language and philosophical position of multiple research paradigms.

References

Bridgman, K. E. (2000) Rhythms of awakening: re-membering the her-story and mythology of women in medicine. PhD thesis, University of Western Sydney, Hawkesbury, NSW, Australia.

Burnard, P. (1992) *Writing for Health Professionals: A Manual for Writers*. London: Chapman and Hall.

Denshire, S. (2000) Imagination, occupation, reflection: ways of coming to understand practice. MAppSci (OT) thesis, University of Sydney, NSW, Australia.

Denzin, N. K. and Lincoln, Y. S. (eds) (1994) *Handbook of Qualitative Research*. London: Sage.

Fitzgerald, M. (1997) Ethnography. In *Qualitative Research: Discourse on Methodologies* (J. Higgs, ed.), pp. 48–60. Sydney: Hampden Press.

Goodfellow, J. (1997) Narrative inquiry: musings, methodology and merit. In *Qualitative Research: Discourse on Methodologies* (J. Higgs, ed.), pp. 61–74. Sydney: Hampden Press.

Guba, E. G. and Lincoln, Y. S. (1994) Competing paradigms in qualitative research. In *Handbook of Qualitative Research* (N. K. Denzin and Y. S. Lincoln, eds), pp. 105–117. London: Sage.

Hayward, A. L. and Sparkes, J. J. (1982) *The Concise English Dictionary*. Hertfordshire: Omega Books.

Higgs, J. (1998) Structuring qualitative research theses. In *Writing Qualitative Research* (J. Higgs, ed.), pp. 137–150. Sydney: Hampden Press.

Higgs, J. and Adams, R. (1997) Seeking quality in qualitative research. In *Qualitative Research: Discourse on Methodologies* (J. Higgs, ed.), pp. 82–94. Sydney: Hampden Press.

Higgs, J. and Cant, R. (1998) What is qualitative research? In *Writing Qualitative Research* (J. Higgs, ed.), pp. 1–8. Sydney: Hampden Press.

Higgs, J. and Radovich, S. (1999) Narratives on qualitative research. Paper presented at AQR '99 International Conference: Issues of Rigour in Qualitative Research, 8–10 July, Melbourne, Australia.

Leininger, M. M. (1994) Evaluation criteria and critique of qualitative research studies. In *Critical Issues in Qualitative Research Methods* (J. M. Morse, ed.), pp. 95–115. Thousand Oaks: Sage.

McAllister L. (1998) What constitutes good qualitative research writing – in theses and papers? In *Writing Qualitative Research* (J. Higgs, ed.), pp. 217–222. Sydney: Hampden Press.

McCormack, B. (1998) An exploration of the theoretical framework underpinning the autonomy of older people in hospital and its relationship to professional nursing practice. DPhil thesis, University of Oxford, Oxford, UK.

Morse, J. M. (ed.) (1997) *Completing a Qualitative Project: Details and Dialogue*. Thousand Oaks: Sage.

Smith, D. (1997) Phenomenology: methodology and method. In *Qualitative Research: Discourse on Methodologies* (J. Higgs, ed.), pp. 75–80. Sydney: Hampden Press.

Thorne, S. (1997) The art and science of critiquing qualitative research. In *Completing a Qualitative Project: Details and Dialogue* (J. M. Morse, ed.), pp. 117–132. Thousand Oaks: Sage.

Titchen, A. (2000) *Professional Craft Knowledge in Patient-Centred Nursing and the Facilitation of its Development*. DPhil thesis, University of Oxford, Oxford, UK. Oxford: Ashdale Press.

Index